60-PLUS in Massachusetts

The guide to benefits, bargains, and better living for people over 60.

SECOND EDITION

Priscilla and Victor Claman

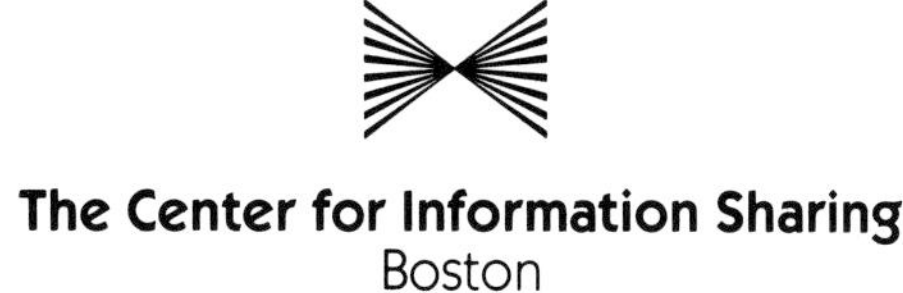

The Center for Information Sharing
Boston

Acknowledgements

Many people have helped us to compile and present the information in this book. Without their interest and cooperation the job could not have been done. In particular, our thanks go to the staff of agencies and organizations who took the time to furnish information and review the material, especially John Flynn, Massachusetts Executive Office of Elder Affairs; Ruth Mendelsohn, Massachusetts Association of Older Americans; and Virginia Robinson, Action for Boston Community Development.

Center Staff

Center for Information Sharing staff who worked with the authors to develop this book included: Jane Lytle, Marcia Sorcinelli, Brigitte Gibson (intern), and Danis Collett, designer. The second edition was developed with the assistance of Jane Hunerwadel and Wendy Bedenbaugh.

Photo credits

We would like to thank all those who provided photographs, particularly the Massachusetts Department of Commerce and Development, Division of Tourism, which furnished most of the photos. Other sources are as follows: The National Park Service, p. iv; Jane Lytle, pp. 3, 29, 39, 51, 22, 90 (U.S.S. Constitution; The Appalachian Mountain Club, Bellerose p. 15, Eugene Skevington (mountain climbing) 70, (canoeing) 70, Bellerose 84; Museum of Fine Arts, p. 8; The Boston Red Sox, p. 11; The New England Patriots, p. 13; The Boston Bruins, p. 13; Drumlin Farm, The Massachusetts Audubon Society, p. 16; The New England Aquarium, p. 18; Old Sturbridge Village photos by Donald F. Eaton, p. 19; Edaville Railroad, Edwill H. Brown, pp. 23, 24; Faneuil Hall Marketplace, Inc., p. 33; Worcester Art Museum, Daniel P. Duffy, p. 34; Museum of Afro American History, p. 14; The Greater Boston Convention & Tourist Bureau, pp. 38, 64, 74, 80, 85; Hancock Shaker Village, p. 54; Peabody Museum of Salem, M.W. Sexton, p. 75; The Museum of Our National Heritage, Hillel Burger, p. 77; Museum of Transportation, Bill Litant, p. 79; The First Church of Christ, Scientist, Herb Franklin, p. 90.

Information Contained In This Edition

We have used our best efforts to assure that the information in this book is correct, but there is no guarantee of accuracy, and the reader should regard the information as subject to change. To check out the current status of programs and eligibility requirements, we encourage the reader to contact directly the agencies and organizations which administer the programs.

SECOND EDITION

For information, address: The Center for Information Sharing
77 North Washington Street
Boston, MA 02114

Library of Congress #85—072738 ISBN #0-939532-01-8

1. Retirement-Massachusetts 2. Pre-retirement planning 3. Personal finances
1. Title 2. Title: Sixty-Plus in Massachusetts 3. Claman, Priscilla and Victor

1 2 3 4 5 6 7 8 9 0

To order additional copies of this book, call (617) 742-3222 or write to the address above.

Contents

Enjoying Massachusetts

Where history was made

Clockwise:

Mayflower II
Plymouth (617) 746-1622

A full-scale reproduction of the ship that brought the pilgrims to Plymouth in 1620. See No. 12, p.65.

Concord Bridge
Concord

Veteran's Day Parade
Taunton

Annual parade celebrating Bristol County's role in the Revolution.

Memorial to the Mohawk Indians
Charlemont

Marks the Mohawk Trail which was used as a footpath by the tribe.

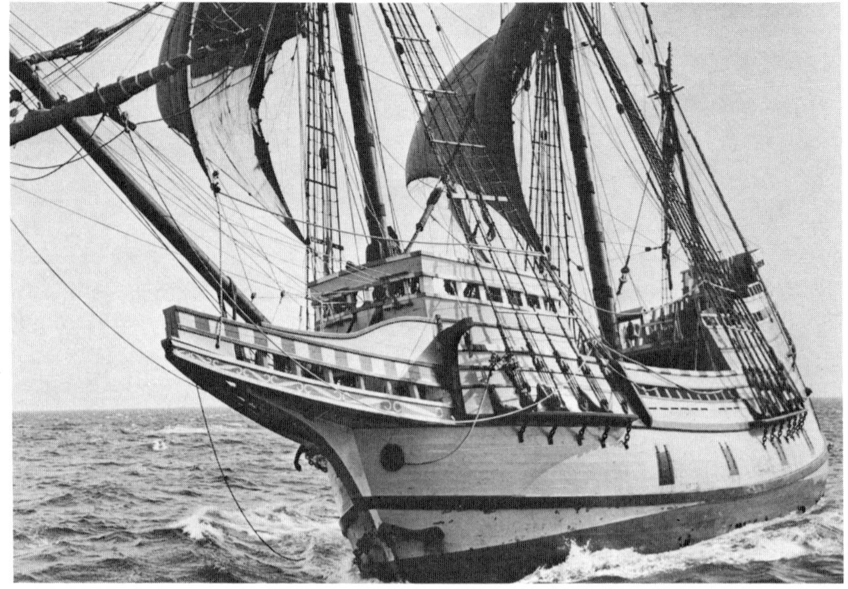

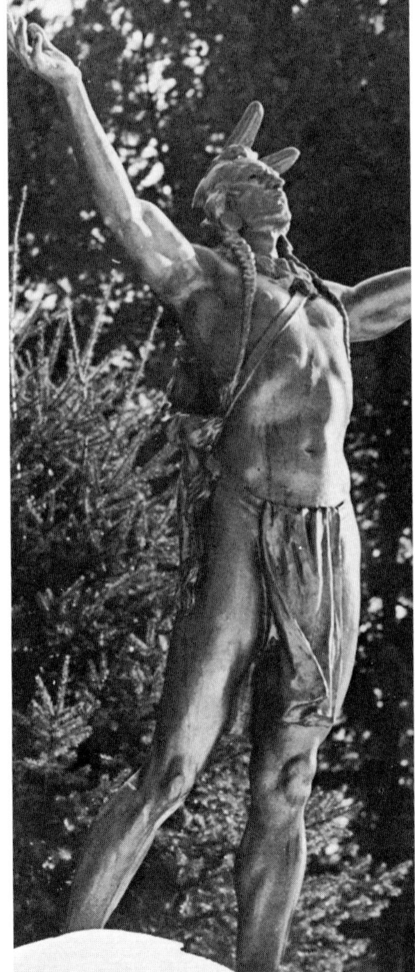

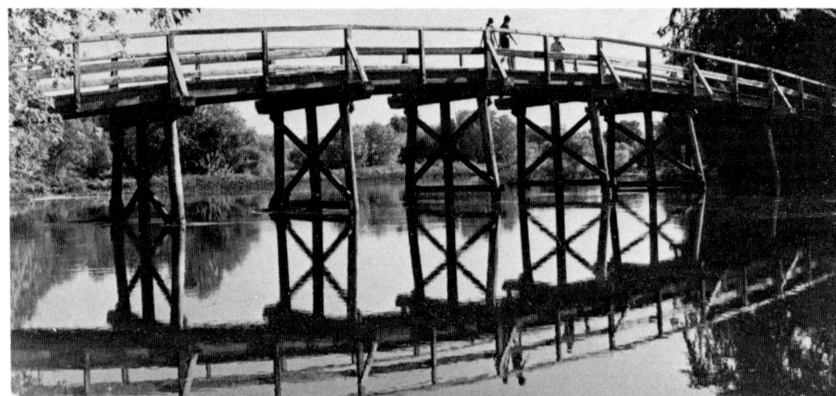

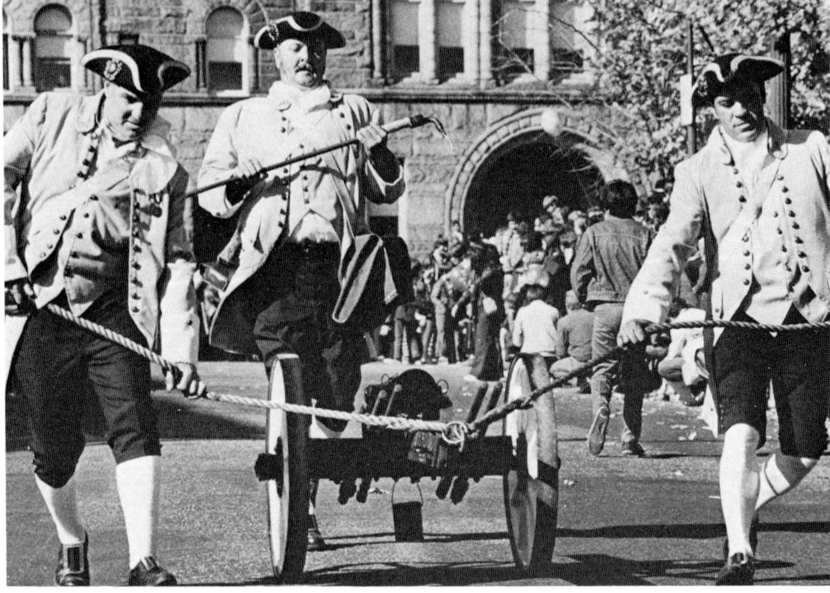

Now You Have the Facts

People in Massachusetts are very lucky—especially older people. Not only are there hundreds of historical and beautiful places to visit, but there are places to get help when it's needed *and* some special bargains reserved specifically for older people.

But to take advantage of all this, you have to know about it. And that's the purpose of this book—to provide you with facts about the special things available to older Massachusetts residents, as well as some helpful hints for a fuller life.

Helping yourself, a friend or a relative

This book is for you

- **if you are 60 or over and living in Massachusetts**
- **if you have a relative or a friend you want to help**
- **if you are planning for your retirement**

Many government agencies and businesses offer special benefits to people 60 and over. This book will tell you what they are and how to get them, and where to complain when things go wrong. You will find some practical advice and maybe some surprises. If not *all* this information is useful to you, it may be useful to a friend or relative. And if there's something we haven't mentioned, look inside the back cover ("Did We Miss Something?") for places to get the information you need.

How to use this book

You may want to read this book from cover to cover or just use it as a reference for the particular subjects of interest to you. There's a detailed table of contents that can be used as an index.

Remember that each section is *not* intended to give you all the details. Rather, we've tried to provide a paragraph or two for general understanding *and* an address or telephone number to call for more information. It's important to get in touch with the agencies or organizations listed, since they are the best sources of detailed information for your personal circumstances and the area you live in. You'll find telephone numbers printed in **heavy type.**

If you live in Boston, there's an extra section—"Boston Page"—on page 90.

Suggest Something for Your Community

You may discover something in these pages—an organization or activity—which doesn't exist just now in your own community but which you think would be a good idea. By all means bring it to the attention of your mayor, selectman, or council on aging (see pp. 81-83). With a little effort, you may be able to launch something new and worthwhile for your community.

How "The System" Works

There *is* a "system," a complex array of government programs and private assistance efforts intended to provide help when you need it. For many people, the most confusing parts of "the system" are the government agencies and programs. Here are the basics of what you'll find in Massachusetts.

In your town or city

At least 330 of the 351 towns and cities in Massachusetts have a department of local government called a **council on aging**. A council on aging is made up of local residents who are dedicated to helping the older people in the community. The council will try to give you the information that you need and may run a club with special programs and special trips or outings. The council will also know which local stores will give you special discounts. In the bigger towns and cities, local councils on aging have offices and run senior citizen centers. You'll find your local council to be an excellent source of information.

Check in the back of this book (pp. 81-83) for the phone number of your council on aging. The councils for the 50 largest communities are listed there. If your community's council is not included, call your town or city hall for the number.

Your state government

Massachusetts has an **Executive Office of Elder Affairs** (EOEA), in Boston. The purpose of this department is to make sure that Massachusetts gets all the federal money it should and that the programs in Massachusetts for older people that use state and federal money are run well. The EOEA will not give you money or services itself, but it does offer information about where to get services and financial assistance.

These are the information numbers:
If you live in the Boston area: **727-8931.**
If you live outside the Boston area:
1-800-882-2003 (toll free).

The federal government

The federal government is the source of most of the money for government benefits for people 65 and over. Some of these benefits come through federal offices in your area, such as the Social Security office. Other benefits come to you through state offices; for example, Medicaid (federal and state money) comes through a welfare office. It is often confusing and difficult to find the right place to get the help you need. This book will help you with that problem.

Tips on how to make the red tape work for you

You might not be used to calling places or agencies that are strange to you, where you don't know anyone. Or, you might feel that you don't like to ask for things or ask for help because you've always tried to handle your problems yourself or with your family. But government is there to serve you, and its programs and agencies can make your life easier. And there are things you're *entitled* to if you're willing to make the effort to get them.

In these days of budget cutbacks, you should expect there to be a lot of forms, questions, and occasional delays. Here are some special hints:

Call first to make sure that you are going to the right place, that the address is still correct, and that someone there will be able to help you.

Bring something to read or a friend to talk to in case you have to wait a while. Some of the larger offices can be very busy.

Ask questions until you understand. The people you meet in government offices are under pressure sometimes, but they really want to help you.

Ask for and write down the name of the person you are talking to. It might be important later. Also, you can give a friend the name of a person who was especially helpful and courteous.

Carry proof of age with you. You will need a driver's license or a copy of your birth certificate when you go to a government office.

Don't ignore or throw out letters you get from government agencies. If you don't understand what they mean (and they can be confusing), ASK! Call the person who signed the letter and make sure you understand, or you could lose your benefits.

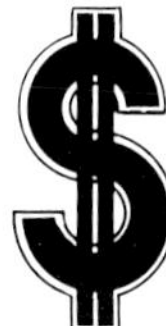

Money Matters

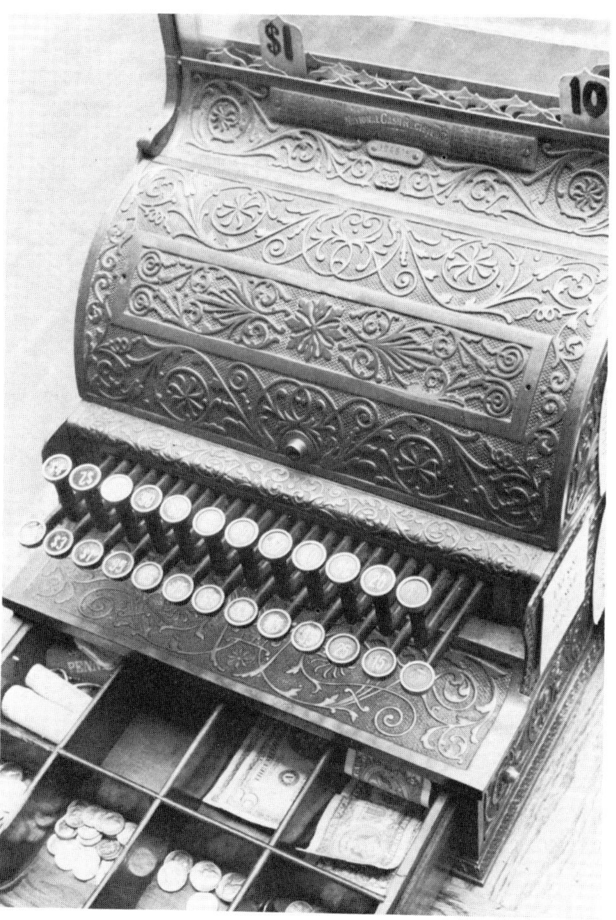

Money is always there but the pockets change; it is not in the same pockets after a change, and that is all there is to say about money.
—Gertrude Stein

If you are among the lucky few who don't need to worry about your shrinking dollars, this section may hold only a few pleasant surprises for you. But for most people who are 60 and older, information about benefits that federal, state, and local government make available will be welcome news. These benefits are not charity; they are the way that our society, through the government, repays older citizens for their contributions to their community and their country during their working years. Local private businesses such as stores and theaters also frequently offer discounts to people who are 60 or over.

In this section you'll find information on:

 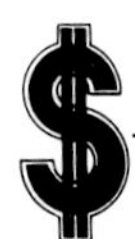

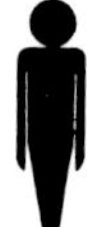

Retirement planning

Many people plan for their retirement by building up investments or savings that will add to their Social Security and pension income. Planning can make the difference between barely meeting expenses and being able to buy a few luxuries and go on trips.

Before you retire you may want to find ways of increasing the income you make on what you have saved. For instance, you may have some 20-year life insurance that will be fully paid up, or savings in the bank that have been yielding lower interest than you could be getting. Your banker, life insurance agent, or investment counselor can help you determine the right thing to do with your money.

Financial planning *in advance* can also be very important if you are going to have a business of your own, do some traveling, move from your present home, or make some improvements in your home either for your own enjoyment or for rental income.

While there are many reasons to plan for your retirement, there are three especially important things to look into *well ahead of time*: the continuation of adequate health services and health insurance coverage; tax planning; and any immediate investment decisions you may have to make. For instance, when you retire you *may* receive a one-time lump sum pension benefit that could mean you have to decide what to do with a large sum of money; clearly, you will want to avoid having to make a major decision at the last moment.

To find out about your future pension, talk to your employer's personnel officer or an official in your union. Some employers have special pre-retirement planning programs. If there is no such program where you work, check your local community colleges. Many of them offer courses specially aimed at money management, tax and financial planning.

Retirement and unemployment compensation. Because of a recent state law, people in most kinds of jobs can *not* be required by their employer to retire at a certain age. However, if there *is* a required retirement age in your present job, and you want to look for another job, you may be eligible for unemployment insurance while you job hunt. If you retire *voluntarily* and then take another job and work for at least four weeks, you may also be eligible for unemployment compensation if you are laid off from your new job for lack of work. Also, if you lost your old job because of a "reduction in force", you may be entitled to unemployment compensation even if you have been given early retirement benefits upon separation.

Generally speaking, an amount equal to half of your Social Security payment and half of most pensions will be deducted from your unemployment insurance benefits, and you will receive the remainder. For any question you might have about unemployment compensation, call the state's Division of Employment Security:

1-800-322-4944 (toll free)

Health insurance. If you decide *not* to retire at age 65, you may have to decide what to do about medical coverage that your employer has been providing. Ask someone in personnel if you will have to make such a decision; it may be a good idea to check on this a full year before your 65th birthday.

Pre-retirement checklist

Check if you've done it.

At least one year before retirement:

- ☐ Check with your employer about retirement benefits and health insurance decisions
- ☐ Plan your retirement

Three months before retirement:

- ☐ Apply for Social Security or SSI
- ☐ Apply for Medicare or Medicaid
- ☐ Apply for Medex or other coverage

After retirement:

- ☐ Apply for Unemployment Compensation, if you are eligible

Social Security— the GREEN check

Social Security is a federal insurance program providing monthly payments for eligible workers and their families when the worker retires, dies, or becomes severely disabled. A green check will be mailed to you or your bank every month. Your monthly checks may be:

1. **Retirement checks:** full payments if you retire at 65, or reduced payments as early as age 62. Higher benefits are available for those who delay retirement past 65.
2. **Disability checks,** if you are a severely disabled worker of any age. You are considered disabled if you have a severe physical or mental condition which keeps you from working and is expected to last at least one year or is expected to result in death. To qualify, you must have worked and had Social Security payments withheld from your paycheck for a certain period of time. If you do not qualify under Social Security, you may be able to get SSI (Supplemental Security Income); see page 7.
3. **Survivors' checks,** for certain members of a worker's family when a worker dies. A lump sum payment can also be made (usually to a widow or widower).

If you have retired or are disabled, certain members of your family can receive benefits: for example, unmarried children under 18 (or 19 if they are full-time students); or disabled children 18 or over who were disabled before 22; or your wife or husband age 62 or over.

Even if you are divorced, if you were married for 10 years or more, you may be eligible for benefits as a dependent of your ex-wife or husband. A divorced and disabled wife who survives a worker to whom she was married for 10 years or more becomes eligible for benefits at age 50. There are many more categories that apply to a worker's dependents.

How to qualify for Social Security

Before you or your family can get monthly retirement benefits, there must be Social Security "credit" for a certain amount of work. In other words, the worker must have contributed to the Social Security fund for a certain period of time. The exact amount of credit depends on age. For example, if you want to get early retirement checks and you reached 62 in 1981, you need 7½ years of work credits; if you reached 62 in 1983, you need 8 years of credits. Anyone who reached 62 in 1984 or later needs 10 years of work credits. Nobody ever needs more than 10 years of work credits to be eligible for Social Security payments.

If both you and your spouse are eligible

If you and your spouse are each entitled to Social Security checks, each of you will receive your own.

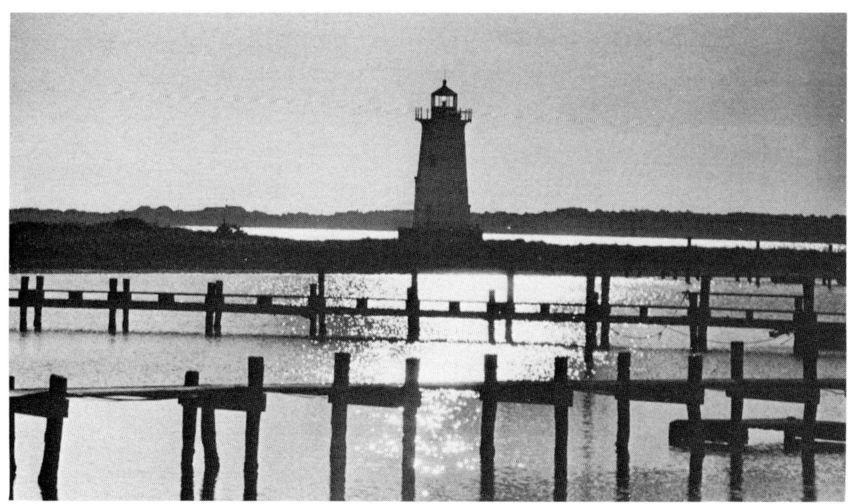

Edgartown Harbor Light
Martha's Vineyard

Once a beacon for whaling vessels, now a welcoming sign to fishing boats and summer tourists.

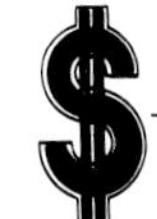

More about Social Security

Estimating your check

The amount of your retirement check depends on your age and your average earnings over a period of years and is calculated according to a special formula. The correct amount will be calculated when you apply for Social Security. But you can estimate what your check will be by asking for a copy of the Social Security leaflet called "Estimating Your Social Security."

If your spouse has died and you qualify for benefits on the basis of your record *and* your spouse's record, you will get an amount equal to the larger of the two earned benefits. For example, if you are over 65 and qualify for $250 a month and your husband was entitled to $300 a month, you will get your $250 *plus* $50.

If you wait to retire beyond 65, you will get 3% more money per month for each year beyond 65, up to 70, that you delay taking Social Security benefits.

Credit for disability is figured differently from credit for retirement checks, but disability checks are also based on former earnings.

Call your Social Security office for help in estimating your benefits.

How much can you earn from working without having your retirement benefits reduced?

As of 1985, if you are 65 or over, you may earn up to $7,320 a year and still receive all your Social Security benefits. If you earn more than $7,320, your Social Security check will be reduced one dollar for every two dollars you earn. If you are over 70, you will receive your full benefits each month no matter how much you earn. Income from your savings, investments or insurance is *not* considered earnings and will *not* reduce your Social Security check.

When to apply

You should apply 3 months before the date when you want to start receiving retirement checks. For disability and survivors' checks, apply as soon as the disability or death has occurred.

Where to apply

To find out where to apply for Social Security, see your telephone directory under "Social Security Administration" for the address and phone number of the office in your area. You may go to the office in person to apply. Or if you are house-bound, call and ask to complete an application over the phone. After you have answered the questions, a filled out application will be sent to you to sign and return to Social Security.

What you should take with you when you apply for Social Security:

1. Evidence of your birth—birth certificate (which you can get from the town or city hall in the place of your birth) or baptismal certificate
2. Your Social Security card
3. The W-2 tax form for the last year you worked (if you are self-employed, a copy of your last federal income tax return)
4. Your marriage certificate, if you're applying for wife's or widow's, husband's or widower's benefits
5. The death certificate, if you are applying for survivor's benefits
6. If you are applying for disability benefits, you should have a letter from your doctor and must know the doctor's name, address, and phone number and the dates you were seen by the doctor.

IMPORTANT: Social Security is complicated. There are many categories and the rules change. You may be entitled to payments, or to larger payments than you are now receiving. Don't get discouraged. Talk to the people at your Social Security Administration office, tell them all the facts, and then be persistent until you feel you are receiving all the benefits to which you are entitled.

Supplemental Security Income (SSI)— the GOLD check

Supplemental Security Income is a federal program that pays monthly checks to people in financial need who are 65 or older and to people in financial need at any age who are blind or disabled. Massachusetts adds to the amount that the federal government provides. A gold check will be sent to you or your bank every month.

The maximum monthly SSI check* that a Massachusetts resident 65 or over can receive is:

- $453.82 for a single person
- $689.72 for a couple

Some people get less than this because they have other sources of income or have a different living arrangement. People who are blind or disabled will get a different amount of SSI; they should check with their Social Security office for details.

You can get SSI even if you have never worked.

You can have some assets and still get SSI. A person who is single can have assets worth up to $1,600 and still get checks. The amount for a couple is $2,400. Assets include savings accounts, stocks, bonds, jewelry, and other valuables a person or couple own. Your house, personal effects or household goods do *not* count as assets in most cases. A car or certain types of insurance policies may not affect your eligibility either, depending on their value.

*As of January 1985

You can earn a little money and still get SSI. People who work while they are getting SSI can earn as much as $65 in a month without any reduction in their SSI checks. After that, the check is reduced $1 for each $2 in earnings over $65 in a month.

You can also have some unearned income. Unearned income includes Social Security, interest on savings accounts, dividends, veterans compensation, worker's compensation, pensions, annuities, gifts, and other income. The first $20 a month in unearned income generally does not reduce the amount of the SSI check.

For eligible people who live in someone else's household—in a relative's house, for example—the SSI check may be reduced.

How to apply for SSI

To apply for SSI, call the Social Security Administration number in your phone book and tell them you're interested in applying for SSI. The person on the phone will ask you a set of questions. You will get a postcard telling you whether or not you qualify, and, if you do, what to bring with you when you come in to fill out the application.

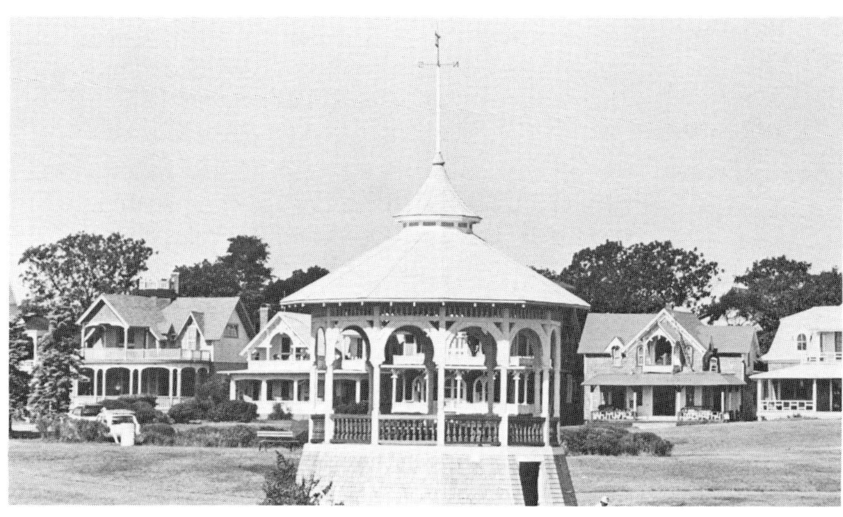

The Bandstand at Oak Bluffs
Martha's Vineyard

The bandstand is surrounded by ornate Victorian "gingerbread" cottages.

 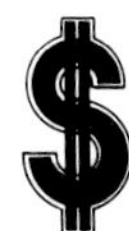

The differences between Social Security and SSI

Social Security	SSI
• a GREEN check	• a GOLD check
• for people who have worked and contributed a sufficient amount to the Social Security fund, and for their immediate families	• for people who have low income, and who are 65 and over or who at any age are blind or disabled
• can provide retirement benefits as early as age 62	• provides income for people who cannot work or who are earning a *very* small amount of money
• can provide disability benefits which are based on salary when working	• can provide disability benefits which are fixed, based on the disability (no previous earnings necessary)
• can provide survivors' benefits	• does *not* provide survivors' benefits
• the Social Security program includes Medi*care* insurance, which can cover a portion of medical and hospital costs	• the SSI program includes Medic*aid* medical insurance, which covers *all* of certain medical and hospital costs
• if you receive Social Security, you are *not* entitled to lower utility rates	• a head of household or principal wage earner receiving SSI *can* get lower utility rates
• you apply for Social Security at the Social Security Administration office nearest you	• you apply for SSI at the Social Security Administration office nearest you

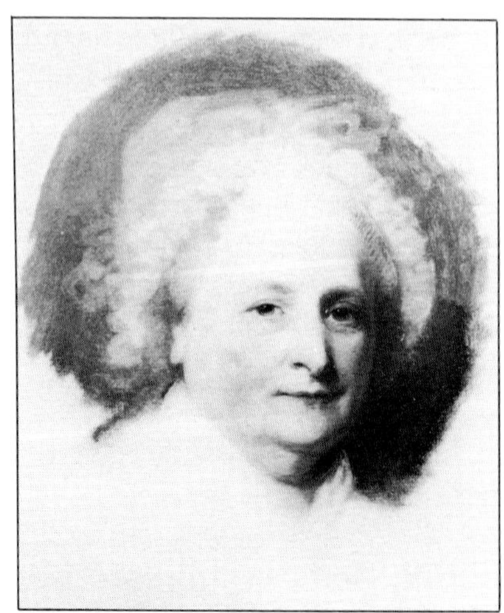

See No. 26, p.66.

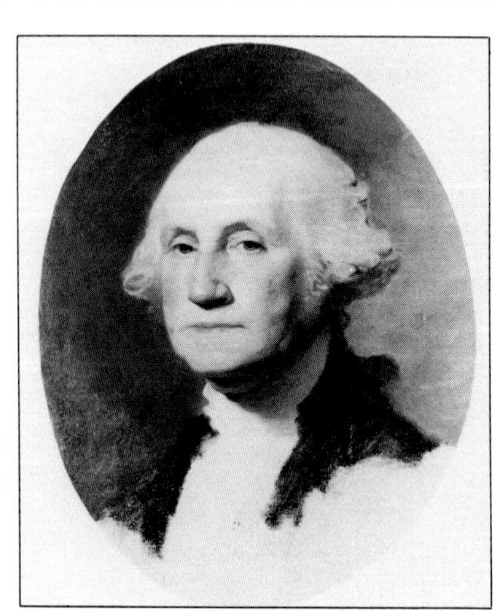

General tips on applying for Social Security or SSI

- You can get help over the phone, but you may have to call several times to get a free line at large Social Security offices. The best times to call are early in the afternoon and late in the month.
- Be sure to ask questions until everything is explained to you clearly.
- If you go in person to your Social Security office, you may have to wait. Bring something to keep you busy, and some food, too. If you don't speak English well, it's best to bring an interpreter with you.
- Bring any letters that you have received from Social Security when you go to their office.
- If you are unable to work any longer and are applying for **Disability**, under either Social Security or SSI, you must know your doctor's name, address and phone number, and the dates when you were seen; and you should have a letter from your doctor.
- Don't ignore any letter from Social Security; if you don't understand what it means, call the person who signed it. Your claim can be denied on grounds of "lack of cooperation" if you don't respond to a letter.
- Collect all the information and documents you will need. A single missing item can mean a delay in getting your benefits.
- Apply within whatever time limits have been set by the Social Security Administration.
- One last tip: Always write down the name of the person you talk to.

About complaints and checks

Complaints about Social Security and SSI

If you need to make a complaint about your Social Security coverage or benefits, you can find out how to do it on page 66.

What to do if you lose your check

Call your Social Security office and give your name, address and Social Security number. They will send you a new one.

How to get your check sent directly to your bank

Your Social Security check or SSI check can be deposited directly to your account. This saves you time and trouble, and this way your check cannot be lost or stolen.

Most banks offer this service—but call your own bank first to make sure. You can have your checks deposited directly in either a checking or a savings account, and there is *no charge* for this service. To get things started, you will have to go to the bank, see a bank officer, and fill out a form. You have to bring a Social Security check with you. The bank will send the application form in to Social Security, and it will take about 2 months before your checks will begin being directly deposited. Until your new depositing arrangement has been set up, you will continue to receive your checks at home.

Banks must cash your check

A recent state law requires that all Massachusetts state-chartered banks honor and cash Social Security, SSI, and retirement benefit checks from the federal government and from any unit of state or local government in Massachusetts.

You need to be a Massachusetts resident and must select a single bank where you will cash your checks. You do *not* need to have an account at that bank, however.

Each time you cash a check you will have to show an identification card that has been issued by the bank. Ask the bank for a form to fill out to get your card. It may take up to one month before the bank can give you your card, and the bank is allowed to charge you a one-time fee of up to $5 to process your application.

Enjoying Massachusetts

Special events

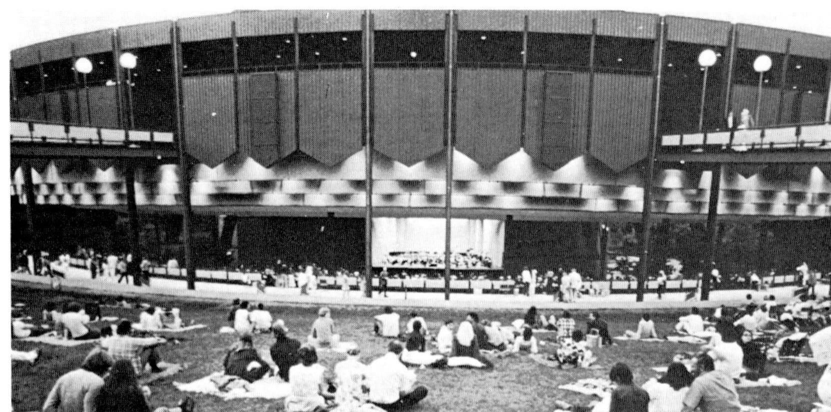

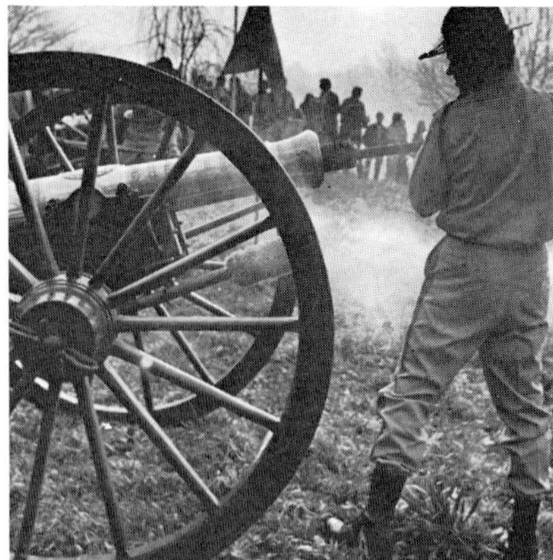

Clockwise from top left:

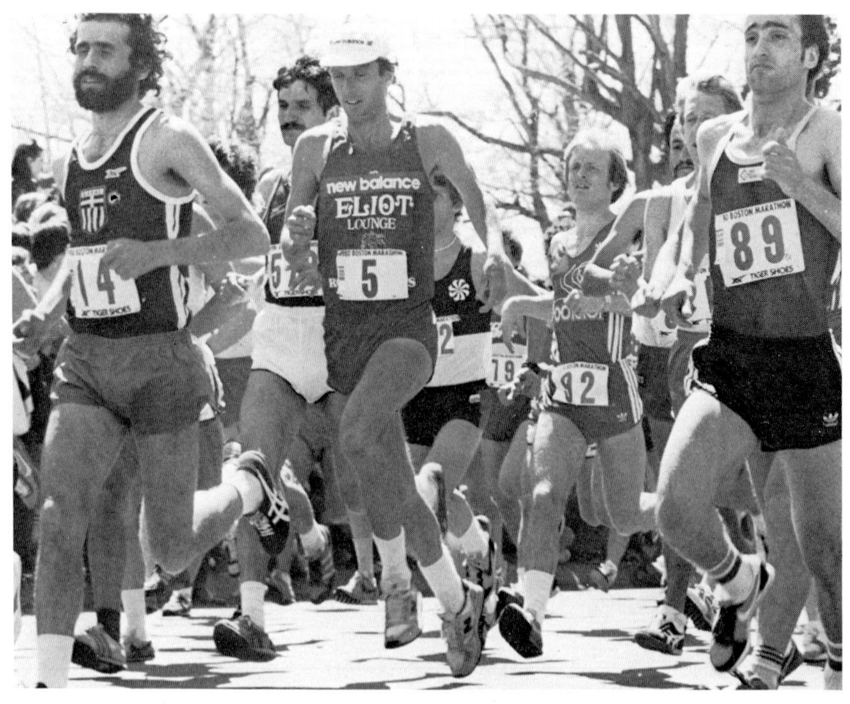

Tanglewood
Lenox (413) 637-1940
Summer home of the Boston Symphony Orchestra and the Berkshire Festival. See No. 74, p.68.

Patriot's Day, April 19th
Concord
Annual re-enactment of the shot in 1775 that was "heard 'round the world."

The Boston Marathon
Every spring thousands of spectators crowd the streets of Boston and its suburbs to watch while thousands of runners take on the famous Boston Marathon.

Hatch Memorial Shell
Boston
Free summer evening concerts on the Charles River played by members of the Boston Symphony.

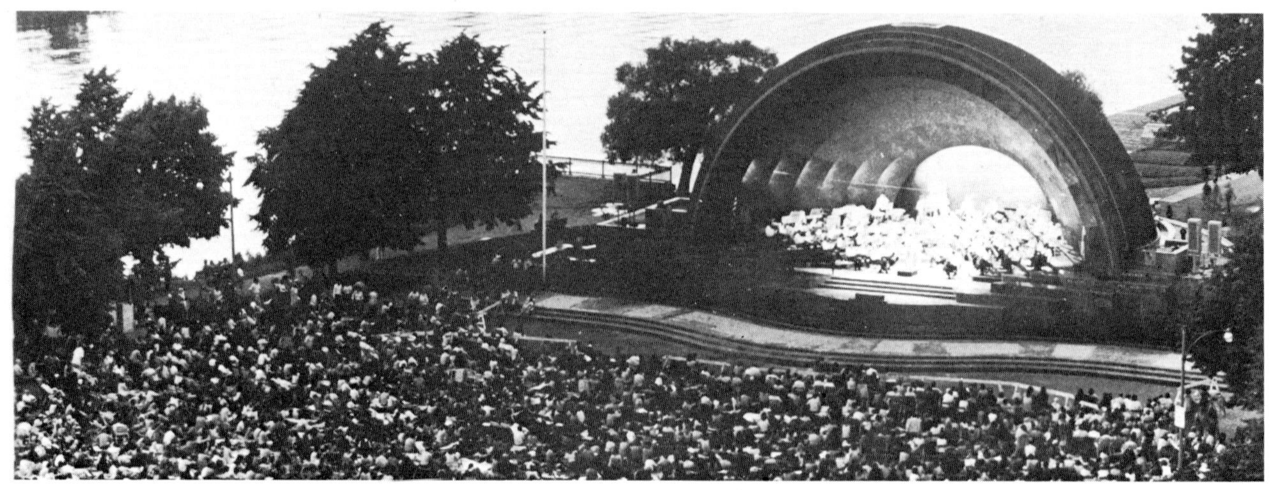

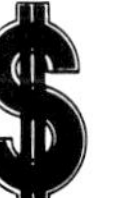

Medicare, Medex and Medicaid: paying doctor and hospital bills

Medicare and **Medicaid** are two different medical insurance programs that help pay for health care:

Medi*care* is a health insurance program run by Social Security for people on Social Security who are 65 and older and for some people under 65 who are disabled. Medicare pays a portion of some medical expenses.

Medi*caid* is a medical insurance program for people receiving SSI and for other low income individuals. It is run by the Massachusetts Department of Public Welfare through your local welfare office. For people who are covered by the program, Medicaid pays the entire amount for most medical expenses.

Medicare

Anyone can be covered by **Medicare** who is:

- 65 and eligible for Social Security (see p. 5)
- under 65 but has been receiving Social Security disability benefits for 2 or more years, or
- under 65, insured under Social Security, and in need of treatment for kidney failure

Medicare has two parts: **hospital insurance** (called Part A) and **medical insurance** (called Part B). The hospital insurance is free to most eligible people; there is a small monthly premium to pay to get the medical insurance. People 65 or older who haven't worked long enough to be entitled to Medicare hospital insurance can buy the protection.

To find out whether you qualify for Medicare and to make sure that you are covered when you reach 65, check with the Social Security office nearest you **three months before you will be 65.**

If you need to make a complaint about your Medicare coverage or benefits, you can find out how to do it on pp. 77-78.

Medicare hospital insurance (Part A)

Your Medicare **hospital insurance** (Part A) helps pay the cost of the following care:*

- Up to 90 days of inpatient care in any participating hospital in each benefit period. (A "benefit period" starts the first time you

*As of May 1985

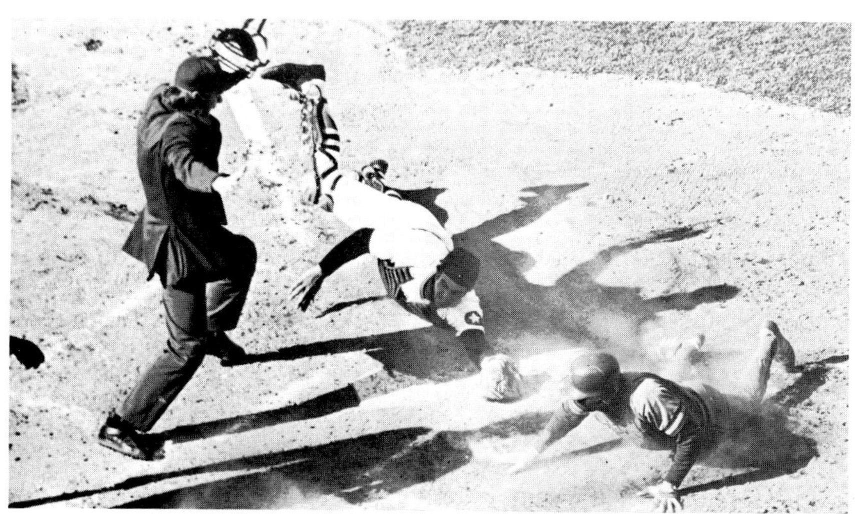

The Boston Red Sox let one get by at Fenway Park, Boston.

 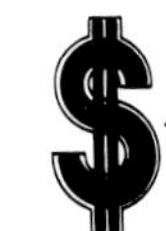

enter a hospital after your hospital insurance begins. The period ends 60 days after you have been out of a hospital or health care facility and are not receiving skilled care. There is no limit to the number of benefit periods you can have.) For the first 60 days, Medicare pays for all covered services except for the first $400. For the 61st through the 90th day, it pays for all covered services except for $100 a day. Care in a psychiatric hospital has a lifetime limit of 190 inpatient days.

- A "reserve" of 60 additional inpatient hospital days. You can use these extra days if you ever need more than 90 days of hospital care in any benefit period. Each reserve day that you use reduces permanently the total number of reserve days that you have left. For each additional day that you use, Medicare hospital insurance pays all but $200 towards covered services.
- Up to 100 days of care in each benefit period in a participating skilled nursing facility. Call Social Security to find out more about this coverage.
- An unlimited number of home health visits from a home health agency after the start of one benefit period and before the start of another. Call Social Security to find out more about this coverage.

Medicare medical insurance (Part B)

If you are eligible for Medicare hospital insurance, you can buy **medical insurance** for very little ($15.50 a month as of January 1985). Unless you say that you *don't* want it, you will automatically be enrolled for medical insurance and charged for it when your hospital insurance begins.

Medicare medical insurance helps pay for the following services:*

- Physicians' services no matter where you receive them in the United States.
- Outpatient hospital services for diagnosis and treatment in an emergency room or outpatient clinic in a hospital.
- An unlimited number of home health visits each year.
- Outpatient physical therapy or speech therapy.
- Other services prescribed by your doctor.
- Hospice care

*As of May 1985

How much does medical insurance pay for? Each year, as soon as you have paid $75 (the annual deductible) for covered medical expenses, Medicare will pay *80 percent* of any additional charges for medical services covered in the policy.

For more information about coverage or if you have any questions about Medicare, call your local Social Security office.

Supplemental insurance

Since Medicare doesn't cover everything, you probably will want some kind of supplemental or "medigap" insurance.

Medex.

Blue Cross and Blue Shield of Massachusetts, private insurance providers, offer special insurance called **Medex** to pay the deductibles and coinsurance not covered by Medicare and to provide hospital coverage, after Medicare stops paying, up to 365 days. There are three separate Medex plans available, offering differing amounts of coverage.

You must have both Part A and Part B of Medicare to be eligible, and the program is only open to new subscribers during a special time of year, usually in April.

For more information
call: **(617) 956-4000**
or write: **Medex**
Blue Cross and Blue Shield
100 Summer St.
Boston, MA 02110

New England Patriots
Foxboro
The Patriots on home turf.

The Boston Bruins score a goal at the Boston Garden.

Other supplemental insurance.

Medex is one of many supplemental insurance programs available to you. You may also want to check the cost and the provisions of the supplemental insurance offered by other private insurance companies. You may be able to save on the cost of the insurance if you can get it through some group or organization you belong to—but make sure the coverage provided is what you need.

HMOs: insurance *and* services

An alternative to "medigap" insurance is one of the HMO (health maintenance organization) programs for senior citizens. An HMO is an organization to which you belong and pay a monthly fee (presently from about $15 to $35, depending on the HMO). In return you get both supplemental health insurance *and* health services.

HMOs are designed to provide coordinated, comprehensive and, as much as possible, preventive care. Although each HMO operates somewhat differently, the health services you get through any HMO are provided by doctors, hospitals, skilled nursing facilities, and home health care services that are designated by or associated with that HMO. Except in emergencies, you *must* use the resources of the HMO; if you use doctors or facilities *not* associated with the HMO, the expenses will not be covered by your membership fee.

There are several different types of HMOs; altogether, 24 HMOs serve most of Massachusetts. Some now have plans for senior citizens; most are expected to have such plans soon.

To be eligible to join, you must live in the HMO's service area, have Part A and Part B of Medicare, and not have end-stage kidney disease. For more information and a list of HMOs:

Executive Office of Elder Affairs
38 Chauncy Street
Boston, MA 02111
(617) **727-4092**
1-800-882-2003 (toll free)

You may also be interested in a publication on HMOs:
More Health for Your Dollar—PF 3270/984
Single copy free from:
American Association of Retired Persons
1909 K Street NW
Washington DC 20049

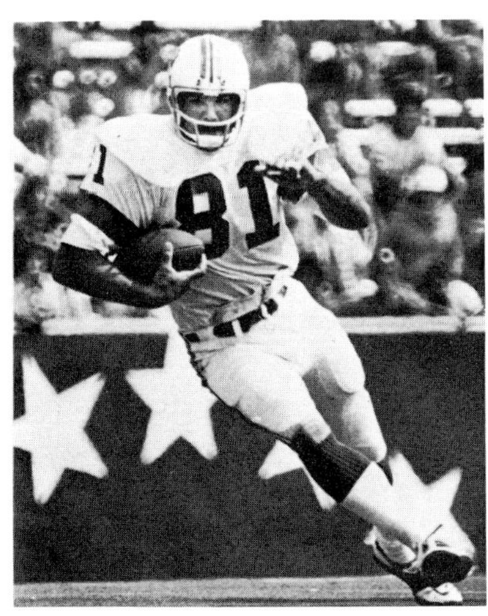

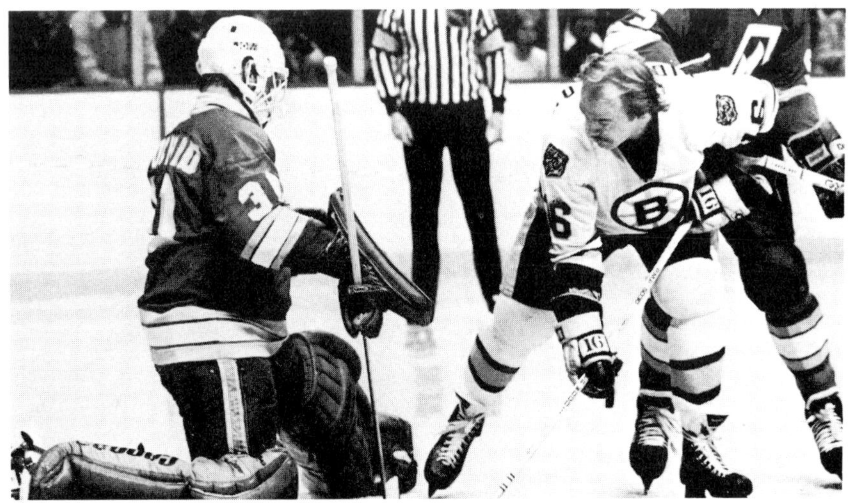

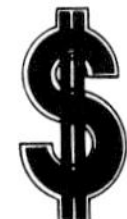

Medicaid

Medicaid is a medical assistance program for needy and low-income people. Any person receiving SSI is *automatically* covered by Medicaid.

Contact your local welfare office to see if you are eligible, or call **1-800-882-1223.** You can find the welfare office nearest you by looking in your phone book under "Welfare" or under "Massachusetts, Commonwealth, Public Welfare."

Medicaid pays for:

- Doctor's fees
- Inpatient or outpatient hospital care
- Laboratory and X-ray charges
- Care in a skilled nursing home
- Adult day care (under certain circumstances)

The other services Medicaid pays for change from time to time. Medicaid may cover such things as dental care, prescription drugs, hearing aids and eyeglasses. Ask at your welfare office.

Can you have both Medicare and Medicaid?

Yes. If you have Medi*care* and a low enough income to qualify for Medi*caid*, you can get a Medicaid card. Many of the expenses that are not covered by Medicare will then be paid for by Medicaid. Ask for the Medicaid person at your local welfare office.

Confused?

SHINE may be the answer

It can be difficult to figure out just what to do as far as getting adequate health coverage is concerned. Recognizing this, state government has started to train volunteers who will work with local councils on aging to help people understand the different alternatives, benefits and costs. The program is called **SHINE**—Serving Health Information Needs of Elders.

Starting in the Lawrence/Andover, Cape Cod, and Middleborough areas, SHINE is expected eventually to be state-wide. Call your local council on aging (pp. 81-83) to see if there is a SHINE volunteer you can talk with or a group session that the council may be scheduling for you and other seniors. If you would like to train to be a SHINE volunteer yourself, see p. 37.

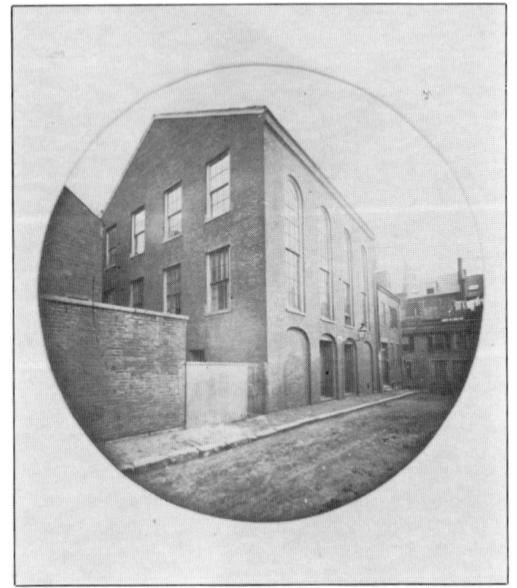

The African Meeting House
Boston

The oldest black church building still standing in the United States. You can see it on the Black Heritage Trail through Beacon Hill. Call (617) 445-7400 for maps and information.

Veterans' Benefits

Veterans' Benefits

The V.A. (Veterans Administration) provides a wide variety of important benefits to eligible veterans and in many cases to the surviving spouse and children and sometimes to parents of the veteran. The benefits may include:

- Pension
- Disability compensation
- Home loan guaranty benefits
- Preference for civil service jobs
- V.A. medical care and hospitalization (veteran only)
- Alcohol and other drug dependence treatment
- Life insurance
- Burial benefits ($150 or more)
- Spouse's pension or dependency compensation

Some benefits are dependent upon there having been a service-related disability. The most important benefits to look into that need not necessarily be service-related are: hospitalization; pension; home loan guaranty; and burial.

The best way to start finding out about eligibility for various benefits is to call the V.A. (you can do this toll free from anywhere in Massachusetts). For yourself or for the deceased veteran in your family, you should be able to tell the V.A.: the veteran's full name and date of birth, branch of service, Social Security number, and dates of service.

If you are a surviving spouse, child or parent of a veteran, you should be sure to check on the availability of benefits *to you.*

For every city and town in Massachusetts there is a Veterans' Agent who can help you to understand and apply for available benefits. Some agents cover several towns. Call your town or city hall to find out this person's number, or call the toll free number below. The Boston and Springfield offices can also give you information and assistance:

Veterans Administration
JFK Federal Building
Government Center
Boston, MA 02203
(617) **227-4600**
1-800-392-6015 (toll free)

Federal Building
1550 Main Street
Springfield, MA 01103
1-800-392-6015 (toll free)

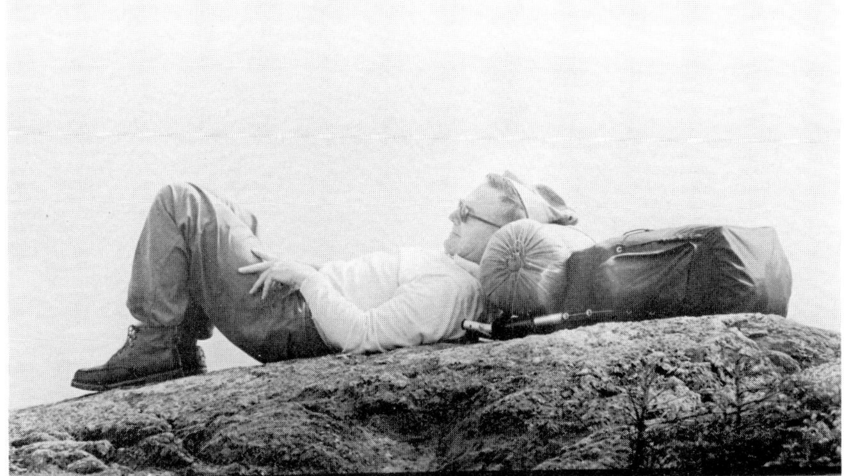

Ah . . . this is the life. Enjoy hiking in one of Massachusetts' many state parks and forests (see p. 62).

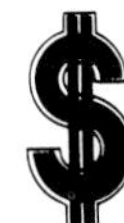

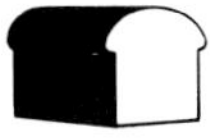 Food Stamps

Food Stamps are coupons used like cash to buy food. Most food stores accept Food Stamps as payment. You may be eligible for Food Stamps depending on the size of your household and your income level. To get Food Stamps you must apply for them through a welfare office and pick them up at the place in your area which distributes them.

First, you must fill out an application. Call the Food Stamp Hotline, toll free, **1-800-882-1223.** The people at the hotline can tell you whether or not you should apply. They can also send out application forms in the mail and give you the address and phone number of the welfare office nearest you. You will need to take the application to the welfare office. Sometimes, if it's hard for you to get to the office, the welfare office will let you mail in the application and then will interview you on the phone. Call them first to find out. If you live in a rural area, you can call your agricultural extension agent and ask how to get the stamps.

If you qualify, the welfare office will send you a voucher (it's called an ATP voucher) and tell you where to take the voucher in your area to pick up your Food Stamp coupons. The Hotline number can also tell you where to take your voucher near you. After you have qualified, the voucher will be sent to you every month, automatically for a set period of time. You will be told how often you need to re-apply.

You can qualify as a single person if your income (including Social Security) is less than $540 per month.* A couple must receive less than $728 (including Social Security) a month to get food stamps.* These income levels are changed from time to time, so check for current levels.

Food Stamp Outreach Program
600 Washington Street
Boston, MA 02111
1-800-882-1223 (toll free)

*As of May 1985

Free butter, cheese, other food

The federally sponsored **Surplus Food Program** distributes butter, cheese and, frequently, milk and rice. In Boston, the food is given out four times a year.

To qualify, a person must have a limited income or be receiving assistance from one of these government programs: Food Stamps, SSI, Medic**aid,** Fuel Assistance, Welfare, Veterans Aid, AFDC, Head Start, or WIC. If not in one of these programs, total annual income must be no more than $7,875* for a one-person household, $10,575* for a two-person household.

In Boston, ABCD (357-6000) distributes the food. If you live elsewhere, call your town or city hall, council on aging, (617) 770-7280, or **1-800-882-2003** (toll free) to find out which organization to contact.

*As of August 1985

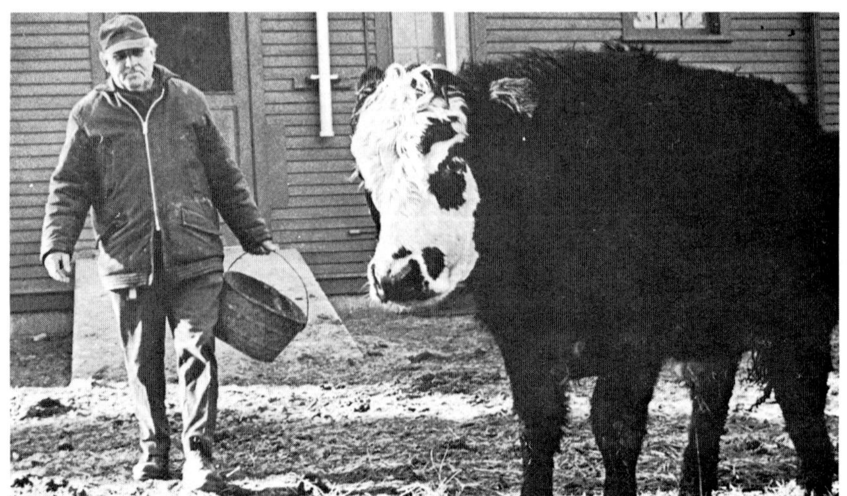

Drumlin Farm/Wildlife Sanctuary
Lincoln (617) 259-9807

The Massachusetts Audubon Society offers teacher- interpreted tours of this 220-acre, turn-of-the-century style farm and wildlife sanctuary. See No. 47, p.67.

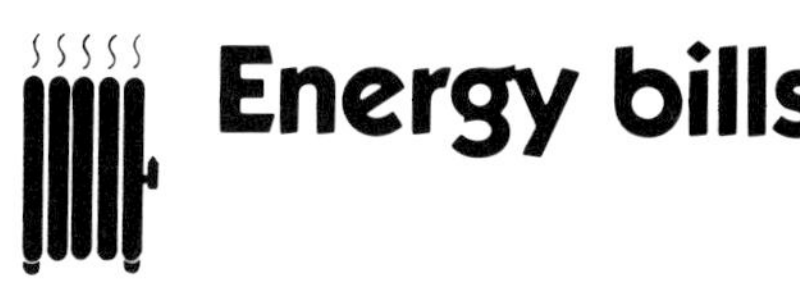

Energy bills

Fuel assistance

Massachusetts is getting Federal money to help people with limited incomes stay warm as fuel costs skyrocket. A significant part of your fuel bill may be paid if you qualify for fuel assistance. To get the number and address of the office in your area that will be taking applications for fuel assistance, call your local council on aging (see pp. 81-83) or:

If you live in the Boston area: **727-8931**

From outside the Boston area:
1-800-882-2003 (toll free)

To qualify for aid, your income must be below a certain level. These income levels may change, so call the fuel assistance office in your area to find out if you qualify. You will also have to show that you can't pay your fuel bills, so save your unpaid bills and any notices you get from the gas or oil company.

If you are unable to apply in person, a home visit may be arranged.

After you apply for aid, it will take several weeks before you will find out if your bill will be paid. If you can't pay the bill during this time, don't worry. Call the fuel company and explain your situation—they will probably be very understanding. If your application for aid is accepted, the money will be sent directly to the fuel company.

If you can't pay your utility bills (gas, electric, telephone), see page 50 for information on what to do.

Save energy/save dollars with home energy conservation assistance

In Massachusetts there are two programs that can help you save energy at home *and* cut your fuel bills: Energy Conservation Service (**ECS**), which is offered through utility companies; and **Weatherization,** which is mostly run by local Community Action Agencies. The ECS program is a comprehensive program for everyone, regardless of income; it involves a home energy analysis called an "audit," and the homeowner or tenants pay for any improvements that they choose to do. Weatherization is only for people who have incomes that fall below certain limits, and the program provides certain weatherization materials and installation free of charge. Here's how the two programs work.

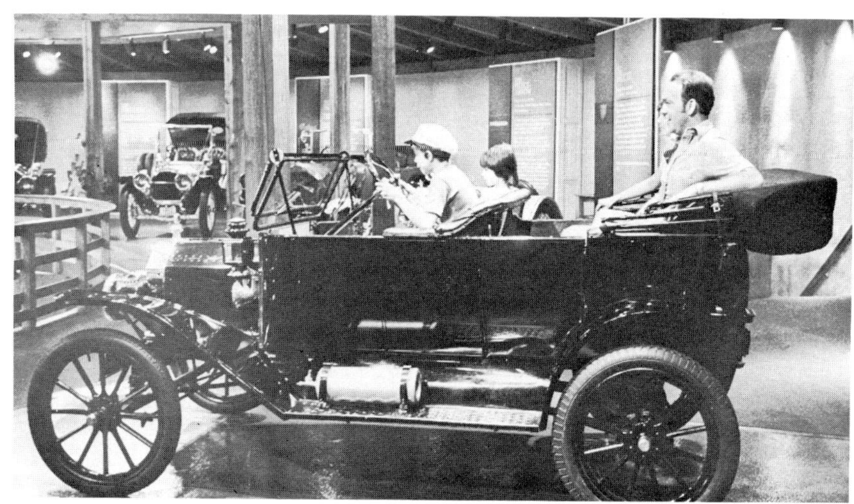

Heritage Plantation
Sandwich (617) 888-3300

Museum of Americana including 34 antique cars, beautiful gardens and trails, military and arts and crafts exhibits. See No. 4, p.65.

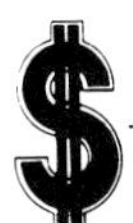

ECS

In many homes and apartments, a few simple steps can make you warmer in the winter, cooler in the summer *and* make your fuel bills lower. To help you take these steps, all utilities are offering assistance, most of them through an organization called Mass-Save.

Call one of the numbers below to arrange to have a *professional energy auditor* visit your home. In most cases there will be a small fee for the audit, but you may not have to pay anything if your income falls within certain limits. The auditor will show you where you are losing or wasting energy. You will be given a written plan that outlines what changes you could make, how much they would cost, and how much energy they would save. You may find out that a single broken pane of glass has been leaking a lot of heat, or that $20 spent on improvements now will save you $100 in the next year alone.

If you decide to follow any of the auditor's recommendations, the auditor will suggest reliable contractors and sources of financing.

Most utilities offer their audits through MassSave. For more information or to request a **MassSave** audit, call (toll free) **1-800-632-8300**.

Fitchburg Gas and Electric and several municipal light departments offer audits themselves. If you are a customer of one of these you can call:

Municipal light departments

Danvers	**774-0005**
Hingham	**749-0134**
Ipswich	**356-4331**
Littleton	**486-3104**
Mansfield	**339-6046**
Marblehead	**631-0240**
Merrimac	**346-8311**
Middleborough	**947-1371**
Peabody	**531-5975**

Fitchburg Gas and Electric

If you live in **Fitchburg: 343-6931**
If you live in **Gardner: 632-5595**

Weatherization: Free home weatherization for lower income people

Improving the energy efficiency of your house—with oil burner adjustment, weatherstripping and caulking around doors and windows, attic insulation, and other weatherization improvements—can help to cut your fuel bills substantially. In Massachusetts there is government assistance for low income people, not only to pay for certain weatherization materials but also to install them. This is called the **Weatherization** program. If you qualify, a trained crew will come to your house or apartment and make energy-related improvements—at no cost to you.

Income limits change from time to time. Recent limits* were $7,875 for a one-person household and

* As of March 1985

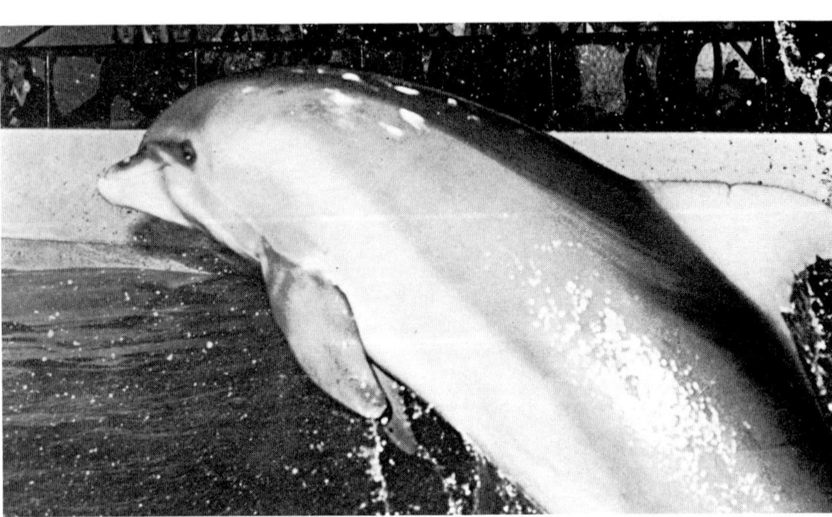

New England Aquarium
Boston (617) 742-8870

Dolphin shows, exotic fish and sea life exhibits, and an enormous central tank. See No. 29, p.66.

$10,575 for a two-person household. If you think you may be eligible, or if you have a question about the income requirements, call your local agency. Any household which has a member who is on SSI is automatically eligible.

The Weatherization program in your area probably is run by your Community Action Agency (there are more than 25 agencies in Massachusetts). To find out the right local number to call, dial either **727-8931** (if you are in the Boston area) or the toll-free **1-800-882-2003** and ask which is the Weatherization office for the city or town where you live. Then call that office and someone there will tell you how to apply and will also arrange for someone to come to your home to see what needs to be done.

For energy conservation information

For more information about such things as insulation, improving your heating system, solar energy, and other ways to save energy dollars without sacrificing comfort, call the energy information service that is maintained by the state's energy office:

Boston area:	**727-4732**
Springfield area:	**739-9615**
Fall River area:	**947-1231, ext. 465**

You may also want to request a free copy of "A Community Guide to Energy Resources" for descriptions of energy conservation assistance programs in your own area.

Water bill discounts

City of Boston

There is a special discount on City of Boston water bills for homeowners who are over 65 or disabled. It doesn't matter if you own a single family house or a triple decker. Houses incorporating space for business use are not eligible. The discount is 15% off each quarterly bill, up to a maximum of $5.00 on each bill. If the water bill is in your name, call for an application form; after you have sent it in, the discount will be taken off your bill automatically. The number to call is: **426-8558**.

Other utility discounts

Heads of household or principal wage earners who receive SSI (see p. 7) are entitled to lower utility rates. For more information, call your utility company.

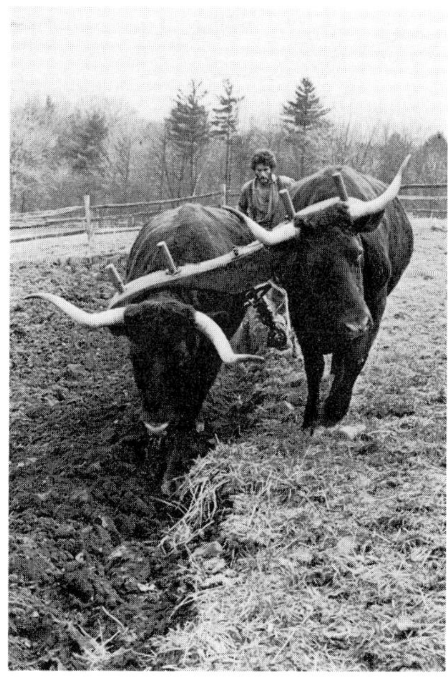

Old Sturbridge Village
Sturbridge (617) 347-3362

A beautiful restored village
See No. 60, p.68.

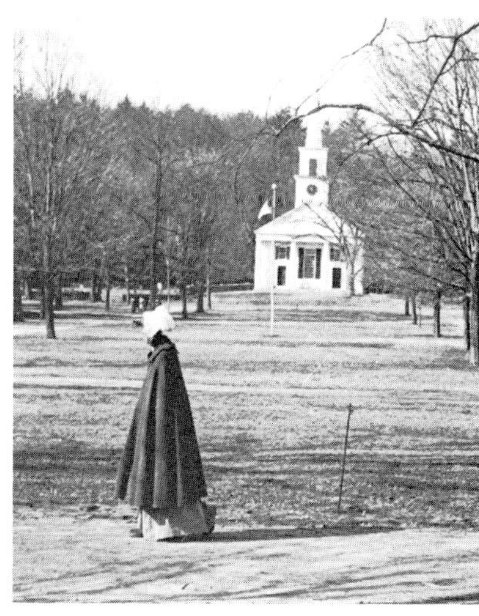

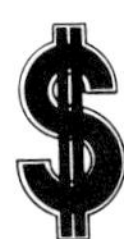

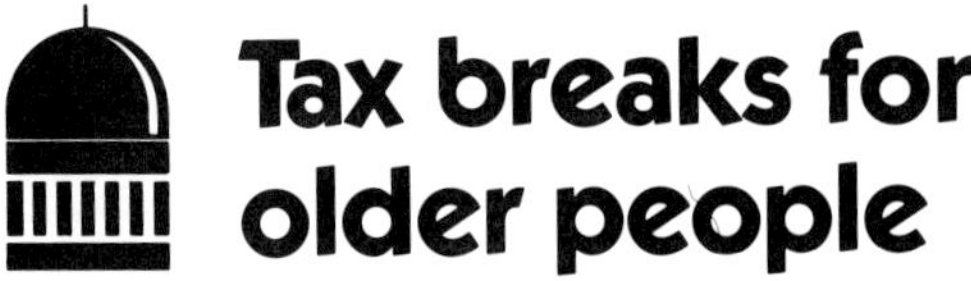

Tax breaks for older people

I'm proud to be paying taxes in the United States. The only thing is— I could be just as proud for half the money.

—Arthur Godfrey

Your federal income taxes

Personal exemptions and tax credits

The Internal Revenue Service offers tax breaks and help with tax forms to older people.

First of all, if you are over 65, you get an **extra $1000 personal exemption.**

In addition, there is a tax credit for some people age 65 or over, depending on their income level. You may claim this credit on Form 1040 and attach a Schedule R, Credit for the Elderly and the Permanently Disabled. The credit also applies to some people under age 65 who retired on a disability pension. If you are married, you and your spouse must file a joint return to claim the credit.

Exclusion of gain on the sale of your home

If you sold your home after July 26, 1978, and were 55 or older before the date of sale, you may exclude up to $125,000 of the capital gain on the sale. In other words, if the value of your house has increased (and that is true for most homes in Massachusetts), you will not have to pay *federal* capital gains tax on up to $125,000 of the difference between what you paid for the home plus any capital improvements you have made, and what you sold it for.

To benefit from the federal tax exclusion, you must have owned and lived in the house or condominium for three of the five years preceding the sale date. You will need to file Tax Form 2119. This is a one-time-only tax benefit—in other words, you can't get another exclusion a year or two from now if you sell another house and have already taken the exclusion. For more information, ask the Internal Revenue Service for Publication 523.

Help filling out the form

If you fill out the first part of the federal tax form (1040, 1040A or 1040EZ) and complete certain line entries, the IRS Service Center will figure your tax and *bill* you for any outstanding amounts due or automatically send you a refund. Information about this free service is in the instruction booklets for Forms 1040, 1040A and 1040EZ.

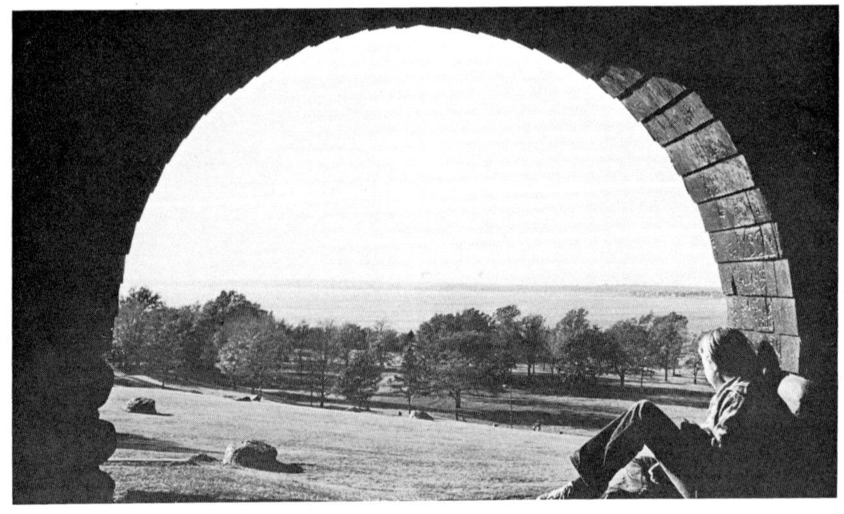

Kennedy Park
Fall River

Looking out from the arched pavilion towards the Taunton River.

Federal tax questions and problems

Your local IRS office is ready to answer your federal tax questions and assist you by showing you how to fill out the forms. Take the forms to them in person, or call:

Boston: **523-1040**
Statewide: **1-800-424-1040** (toll free)
Forms only: **1-800-892-0288** (toll free)

If you have a tax problem that your tax office has been unable to help you solve, write:

Problem Resolution Office
P.O. Box 9103
Boston, Massachusetts 02203

The AARP (American Association of Retired Persons) often has **Tax Aide Volunteers** at tax time to answer questions and help you prepare your return. To find out more, call the IRS, or the AARP in Boston at (617) **426-1185**, or your local council on aging (see pp. 81-83).

Tax breaks publication

For more information about federal tax breaks, you may want to get a free copy of the Internal Revenue Service's publication 554, *Tax Benefits for Older Americans*. Ask your local IRS office, or call or write:

Internal Revenue Service
P.O. Box 25866
Richmond, VA 23260
Toll free: **1-800-892-0288**

State income taxes

You will get an **extra $700 exemption** on your state income taxes if you are 65 or older.

If you are over 55 and sell your home, you do not have to pay capital gains tax on the first $125,000 of gain.

The state tax office in your area will answer questions and help you fill out the forms.

State tax offices:

727-4545	**Boston**
586-4875	**Brockton**
678-2844	**Fall River**
345-0381	**Fitchburg**
774-2740	**Greenfield**
771-2414	**Hyannis**
458-8426	**Lowell**
655-9208	**Natick**
499-2206	**Pittsfield**
744-0210	**Salem**
737-1424	**Springfield**
753-4763	**Worcester**

or call toll free: **1-800-392-6089**

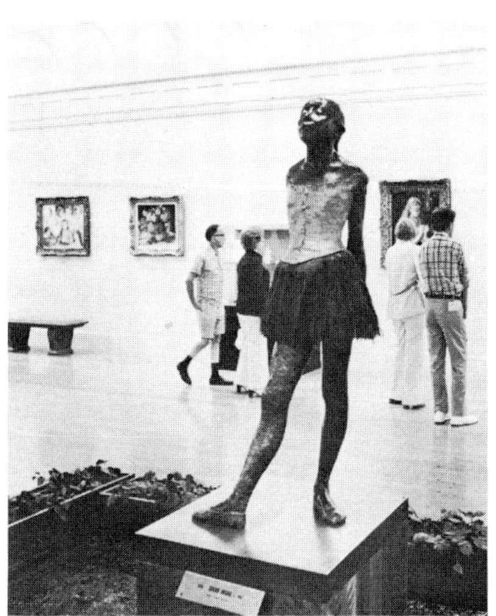

Sterling and Francine Clark Art Institute
Williamstown (413) 458-8109

A strong 19th century art collection including Edgar Degas' sculpture "The Ballet Dancer." See No. 76, p.69.

 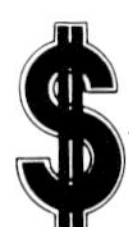

Local property tax relief

There are two kinds of local property tax relief that older people may be entitled to:

- **An exemption**, which is a *reduction* in your tax bill. You do *not* have to repay this at a later date;
- **A deferral**, which permits you to *delay* payment of taxes until a later date. At that time you will have to pay the amount owed, plus interest.

You may be able to get *both* an exemption and a deferral.

Exemptions

Depending upon which provisions of state law your own city or town has adopted, you may be entitled to an exemption of $2,000 to $4,000 on the assessed value of your home or a reduction of from $175 to $500 on your tax bill.

Generally speaking, you or your spouse (if the property is jointly owned) must be 70 or over, have lived in Massachusetts for a period of time, and have limited annual income and assets.

To obtain an exemption, you apply to your local Board of Assessors. An exemption is *not* automatically renewed; you must apply for it every year.

This can be a very valuable benefit for you. Be sure to look into it. Your local Board of Assessors, your Tax Assessor, or someone else in your town or city hall can give you more information. You may also want to get a free copy of *"Property Tax Exemptions for Older Citizens, Surviving Spouses and Minors"* from:

Citizens Information Service
Secretary of State's Office
1 Ashburton Place
Boston, MA 02108
(617) **727-7030**
1-800-392-6090 (toll free)

Deferments

For a deferment (delay) in paying local property taxes, there are also income limitations ($20,000) and other requirements, and a person is eligible at age 65. A deferment is obtained by applying to your local Board of Assessors; contact your town or city hall. The exemptions brochure (above) also contains information.

For more information on exemptions and deferments

In addition to your local assessors and the Citizens Information Service, you can contact:

Property Tax Bureau
Mass. Department of Taxation
100 Cambridge Street, Room 607
Boston, MA 02204
(617) **727-4231**

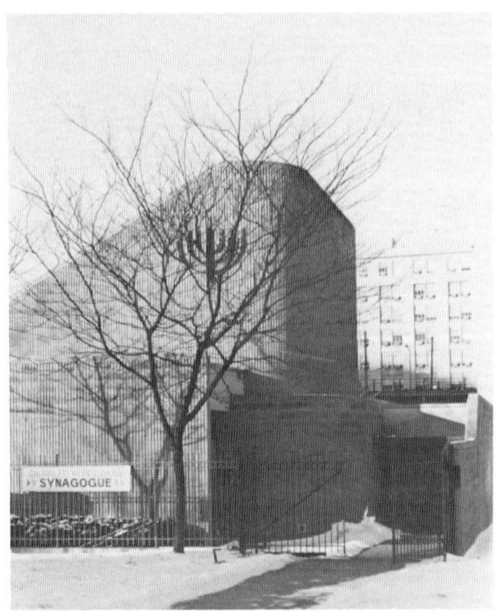

Old and new synagogues in downtown Boston: the modern Charles River Park Synagogue in the West End and the Vilner Shul on Phillips Street in Beacon Hill.

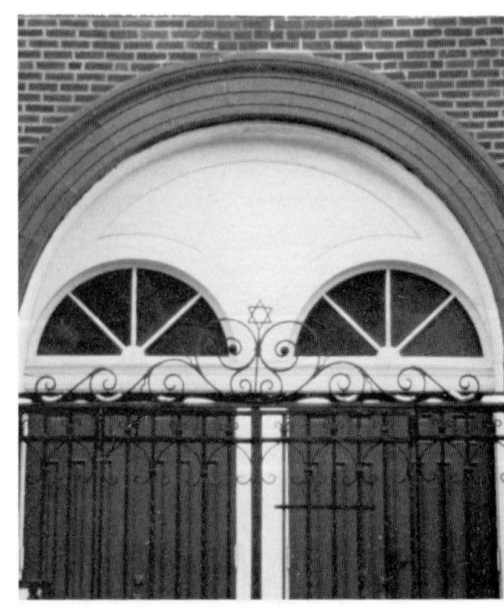

Transportation Bargains

Emergency transportation

Almost all cities and towns have a special vehicle and team to provide free transportation in an emergency. Call your Police or Fire Department.

Intercity transportation

From time to time, some airlines may give special discounts to older people. When planning a trip, be sure to ask the travel agent or airline if any special rates are in effect.

Most large intercity bus companies like Greyhound and Trailways offer a discount from their regular fare to people over 65. But some of the smaller lines do not.

Amtrak offers a 25% discount to people over 65 for any round trip. For conditions and comparative rates, or for special services for the handicapped, call: **1-800-871-7245** (toll free)

Local transportation

Taxi discounts

In some communities such as Cambridge and Boston, there are discounts for older people for taxi rides. Call your council on aging or city or town hall to find out if these discounts are offered in your community.

The special "T Photo Identity Card" for subways, buses, and commuter trains in metropolitan Boston.

If you are 65 or over, and not handicapped, you may ride the **local subway or bus** for 10¢ at all times. If handicapped, you may ride the local subway or bus for 10¢, except from 7-9 a.m. and 4-6 p.m. when you must pay full fare.

If you are 65 or over, or handicapped, you may ride the **MBTA express buses and commuter railroad trains** (the Boston & Maine trains are owned by the MBTA) for one-half fare at all times.

You must have an **MBTA Photo Identity Card** with you to get the reduced rates. You are eligible for the card if you live in the area served by the MBTA. When you go to get your card, you must have with you your birth certificate and a utility bill, or just your driver's license. The card costs 50¢. One place to obtain your card is at the Senior Citizens' Special Needs Office inside the Washington Street subway station (below Filene's) in Boston, Monday through Friday from 8:30 a.m. to 4:00 p.m. The MBTA also visits many cities and towns, spring and fall, to process and issue photo identity cards. Call (617) **722-5438** to find out when they will be in a city or town near you.

If you are a handicapped rider, you must have your physician complete an MBTA medical form. Call (617) **722-5438** to ask the MBTA to mail you a form.

The MBTA publishes a free *Senior Citizens' Reduced Fare Guide* listing all the **discounts for**

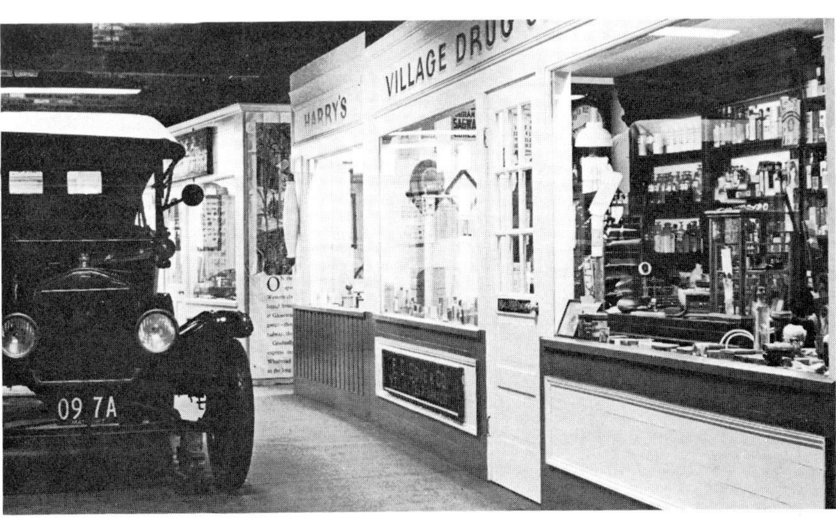

19th century village street
South Carver (617) 866-4526
On the Edaville Railroad grounds.

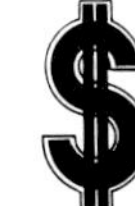

things other than transportation that you can receive by showing your MBTA photo identity card. The listings include museums, stores, theaters and special events, and items such as prescription drugs, hearing aids and eyeglasses. You can pick up your copy at the Washington Street subway station, or write:

MBTA—Sales and Marketing
10 Park Plaza
Boston, MA 02116

Local bus discounts

Most local bus lines run by regional transit authorities offer reduced fares to older people. Often this is a 50% discount. In some cases you will need a special identity card. Ask your bus driver or use one of these phone numbers to get more information about reduced fares.

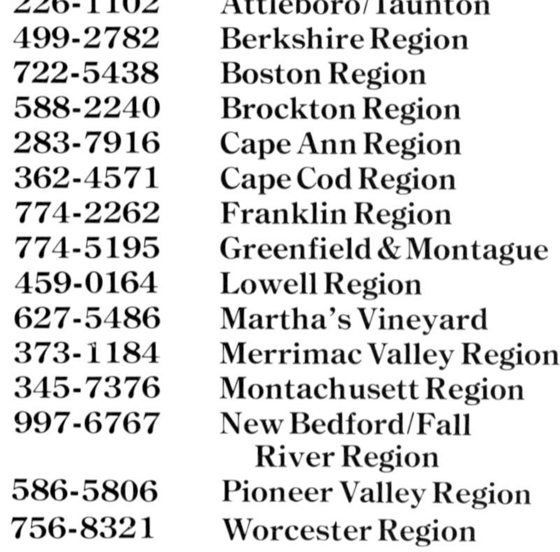

226-1102	**Attleboro/Taunton**
499-2782	**Berkshire Region**
722-5438	**Boston Region**
588-2240	**Brockton Region**
283-7916	**Cape Ann Region**
362-4571	**Cape Cod Region**
774-2262	**Franklin Region**
774-5195	**Greenfield & Montague**
459-0164	**Lowell Region**
627-5486	**Martha's Vineyard**
373-1184	**Merrimac Valley Region**
345-7376	**Montachusett Region**
997-6767	**New Bedford/Fall River Region**
586-5806	**Pioneer Valley Region**
756-8321	**Worcester Region**

Special transportation

The MBTA's **"The Ride"**, for people who can't use regular transportation, is available in fourteen area cities and towns: **Arlington, Belmont, Boston, Brookline, Cambridge, Chelsea, Everett, Malden, Medford, Newton, Revere, Somerville, Watertown,** and **Winthrop**. Tickets are 75¢ one way. To be able to use The Ride, you must have the approval of the MBTA's Office of Special Needs. Phone **722-5123** or **TDD/ TTY 722-5415** for more information.

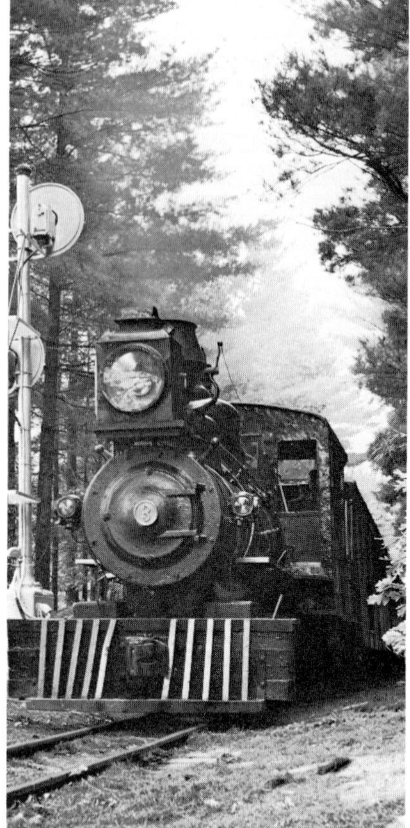

Edaville Railroad
South Carver (617) 866-4526

A 5½ mile steam train ride through cranberry bogs and beautiful scenery. See No. 10, p.65.

Free savings and checking accounts

You may be able to have a bank account that is practically fee-free. The Commonwealth's Commissioner of Banking, pursuant to a recent state law, has ruled that any Massachusetts state-chartered bank which provides one or more of the following accounts—regular N.O.W., regular checking, and passbook savings—must provide for waiver of all fees, charges, and assessments on those accounts under certain conditions. The one exception to the waiver of fees is that the bank may charge up to $5 for each check "bounced" (drawn against insufficient funds).

The law benefits people 65 and over. A bank customer with an individual account must be 65 or over. If it is a joint account, both people must be 65 or over, except that in the case of a married couple one person may be under 65.

For any fee-free account, the customer must ask the bank for a form to fill out, provide evidence of being 65 or over, and request that the fees be waived. It is *not* automatic, even if you already have one of these accounts.

Although not required by law to do so, many federally chartered banks also offer benefits to people 65 and over in connection with certain accounts.

Telephone service

There are no discounts available for older people. However, there *is* protection against cutoff of your telephone service (see p. 50).

There are now separate charges for telephone **service, telephones,** and **long distance.** The least expensive **service** is $4.38 per month; this allows you to make up to 30 "message units" of direct-dial calls a month and to receive an unlimited number of calls. A very local call will cost one message unit for five minutes; a more distant call might cost two, three, or more message units for the five minutes. Additional message units are about 10¢ each. If you do a lot of calling, it might be more economical to have "unlimited" service, which could cost from about $7 to $12 a month.

The least expensive **telephone** you can *rent* from AT&T is about $1.60 a month for a rotary (dial) phone for the wall, desk or table top. This is the rental cost whether it is a newly-installed phone or one you have had for years. Rental includes free replacement if needed. AT&T bills separately for the phones every *three* months; charges are $4.87 for one phone, $9.74 for two phones. Or you may want to *buy* your own phone from a store.

Long distance is a third part of your telephone charges. You choose a "carrier" (company) and are billed on an itemized bill for each call you make. Some carriers have a monthly minimum; others do not.

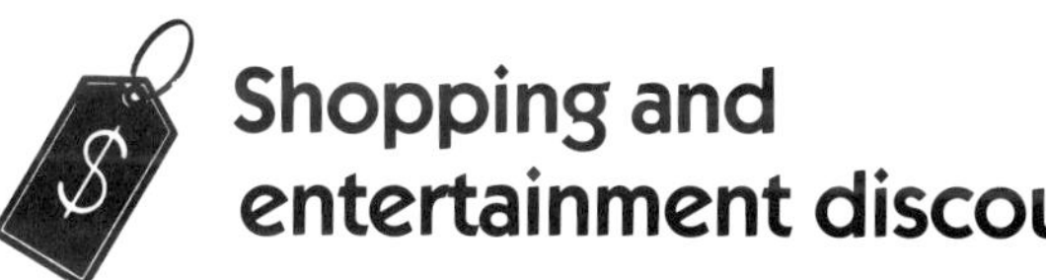

Shopping and entertainment discounts

Stores in your area may offer discounts to older people. Your council on aging may keep a list of such businesses in your community. Call the council (see pp.81-83) and ask which local stores and businesses offer the discounts, how old you must be to qualify, and what kind of proof of age you need. Some councils give out lists of these stores.

"Silver Pages"

In addition to the listing of stores in your area that your local council on aging can give you, you may be interested in a new publication called "The Silver Pages™ Senior Citizens' Discount Directory for the Greater Boston area". Scheduled for publication in December, 1985, by Southwestern Bell Telephone Company, it will include listings of stores, restaurants and many other businesses that make special offers and provide discounts—often 10% to 20%—to people 60 and over. The directory will be free, as will the plastic "Silver Savers' Passport" identification card you must have to get the discounts. Details are available by calling:

1-800-252-6060 (toll free)

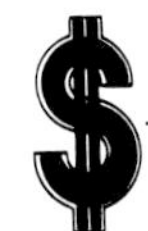

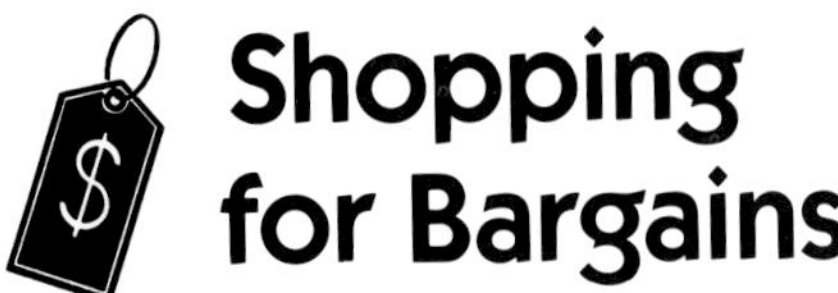

Shopping for Bargains

To be sure, check with your local council on aging to see which stores in your area offer special discounts to people over a certain age. But don't forget that many shopping bargains are available to everyone, regardless of age. All it takes is some time and effort to find the good buys—and you may even enjoy the search, as well as the social aspects if you go with a friend or a group. And of course there's the satisfaction of knowing that you've really gotten a bargain. But *have* you? Ask yourself these important questions before you buy:

- Is it something I really want or need?
- Does it have the features or qualities I want?
- Is it really less expensive than the identical item purchased elsewhere, perhaps closer to home?
- Is the quality acceptable—if the price is lower because it's a second or an irregular or last season's style (although much "bargain" merchandise these days is top quality), is that OK with me?
- Can I really afford it on my budget—it may be a bargain, but are there other things I need my money for?

Sales

Many stores, particularly department stores, periodically reduce inventory by having a sale. Some books, such as the *Guide to Off-Price Shopping* (below), contain lists showing which types of items are likely to be on sale in particular months. Also keep alert for special sales, but beware the "loss leader" item that's put on sale really as an inducement to get you to come into the store to buy other merchandise at regular prices.

Factory Outlets

Sometimes a factory has a retail store at or near the factory. Sweaters and footwear are two typical kinds of merchandise you may be able to buy from such outlets, saving money because overhead is low and you're buying direct. Going to a factory store can be fun, too, and can give you a sense of "connection" with the place where the item was actually made.

Off-Price Stores

You're probably familiar with stores that feature inexpensive items at low prices or specialize in damaged but still serviceable goods. Well, those are *not* "off-price" stores. Off-price stores, which have been increasing in number and sales volume in recent years, sell name-brand merchandise at lower—and sometimes substantially lower—prices. Often they have low overhead with few salespeople, one of the ways they keep prices down. There are many off-price stores—perhaps as many as 300 in Massachusetts—and several Massachusetts-based chains, including Marshall's, T.J. Maxx (Zayre-owned), and Carter's. And of course there's Filene's Basement. For listings of stores and what they specialize in, see the books listed at the end of the section.

Fall River/New Bedford

The biggest concentration of off-price and factory outlets in Massachusetts—perhaps 100 or more—is in the Fall River/New Bedford area. For a free guide, call or write for:

Factory Outlet and Off-Price Outlet Guide
Bristol County Development Council
Dept. 60
P.O. Box BR-976
New Bedford, MA 02741
(617) **997-1250**

If you are a member of a group that would like to visit the area, the Council can assist with group tour planning.

Medicines

If you are taking medication, ask your doctor if there is a generic equivalent you could take instead of a trade-name drug. Generic medicines are less expensive primarily because there are no significant advertising and other promotion costs reflected in the sales prices. In addition to inquiring about prescription medicines, ask your doctor or pharmacist about ways to save on aspirin, vitamins, and similar products; "aspirin", for instance, is a specific chemical compound, and all tablets must meet the same federal standards. Finally, you may want to look into the AARP's non-profit mail order pharmacy service (see p.85).

Buying a new car

These days you should never have to pay the full sticker price—unless the particular car you want is in very high demand and limited supply. Dealers are prepared to bargain with you and, indeed, expect you to try to get the price down. You can get some idea of how much "room" there is in the sticker price by consulting a current copy of Edmund's *New Car Prices,* which shows for each car what a dealer must pay for the car and what the manufacturer recommends as the "list" or "sticker" price (it is the manufacturer's recommended prices which are shown on the sticker on the window). Once you have decided just which car you want, shop around to see which dealer will give you the best price.

If you want to see if you can get the price down really close to the bone, you may want to investigate an "off-price" automobile broker. How this works is explained in the *Guide to Off-Price Shopping* (below).

Membership Clubs and Cooperatives

You may find you can become a member of a club which buys merchandise and then resells it to its members. Often the merchandise is resold in a low-overhead warehouse setting, at prices not much above wholesale. To belong to such a club you have to pay an annual membership fee, so obviously you would want to buy enough in a year so that the savings exceed that fee. Some clubs are open only to people who are employed by or associated with a particular organization, such as a government unit or a credit union.

In your community there may also be a food cooperative you can join. In a cooperative, the big savings usually come from selective bulk buying and from members contributing their own labor to stock shelves and handle checkout counters in order to keep overhead low.

Travel

Air travel costs can be reduced substantially if you have the time and ability to be a stand-by and leave on short notice. As an alternative to staying in a hotel, you may want to consider bed and breakfast in a private home (a number of reservation services are listed in the *Guide to Off-Price Shopping,* below).

For More Information

Successful bargain shopping can really save you money, but you have to know where to look and, in some cases, some special techniques. The following are among the books that may be helpful:

The Underground Shopper's Guide to Off-Price Shopping—Sue Goldstein

The 2nd Underground Shopper—Sue Goldstein

Save on Shopping Directory—Iris Ellis

Factory Store Guide to New England—A. Miser and Pennypincher

Try your local library or bookstore; all are available in paperback.

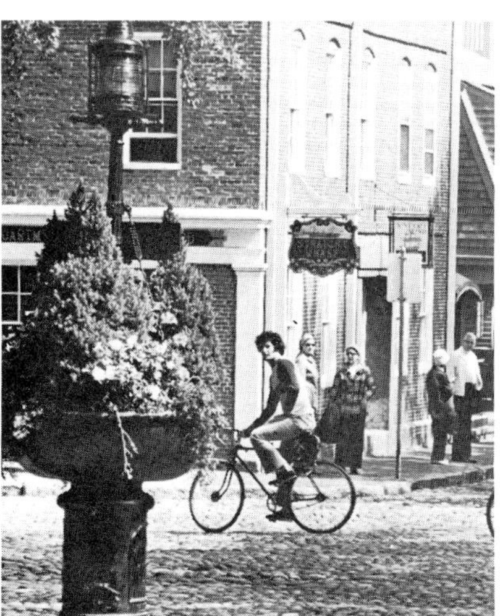

◀ **Center of town**
Nantucket

Cobblestone streets and quaint shops.

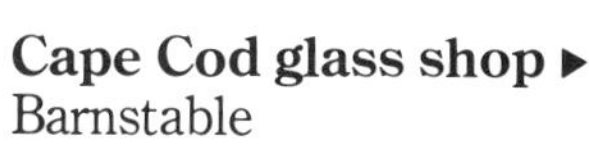

Cape Cod glass shop ▶
Barnstable

Antique glass and reproductions of the New England glass craft.

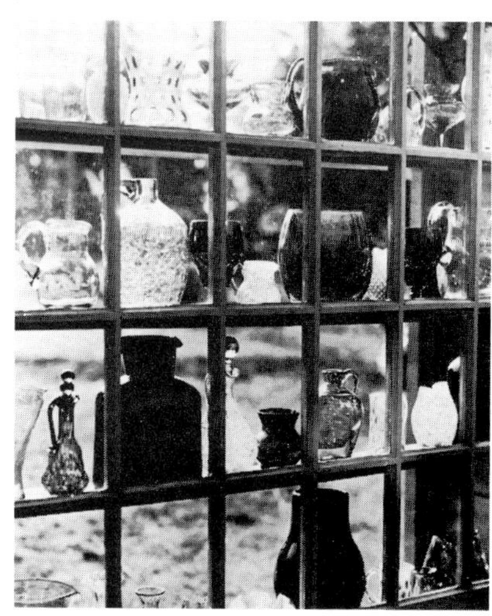

 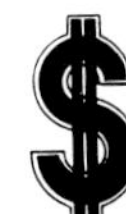

Other money matters

Pension benefits

You are likely to have several options as to how you receive your pension benefits, such as: monthly payments for life or for a certain period of time, or possibly a single lump-sum payment upon retirement.

Choosing the right option *for your particular circumstances* is important for several reasons:

- it is a decision that can*not* be re-made;
- it should be related to your financial resources and to the financial needs of yourself, your spouse, or anyone else who may be going to depend on the pension;
- it will have tax consequences.

Give yourself enough time to make the decision, because there may be some new things to learn about. For example, for a lump sum distribution, for tax reasons one of the things you will probably consider is to put it into a "rollover" IRA (individual retirement account) in a bank. There's nothing especially complicated about a rollover IRA, and your bank or employment counselor can tell you about it, but it may be entirely new to you and you should make sure you have the time to fully understand it.

Money from your home

Your home may be a source of money for you. Obviously, if you sell it and make some other living arrangements, there may be a surplus you can use for other purposes. But there may also be a way for you to "tap into" the equity tied up in your home *without* selling and moving—through **home equity conversion** (for more information, turn to page 47). Or, there may be some income potential if you take in someone to share your home, rent out a room or two, or create an "accessory apartment" (more on p. 40).

Discount/Bargain Index

Here is an index to help you find many of the money-savers in this book.

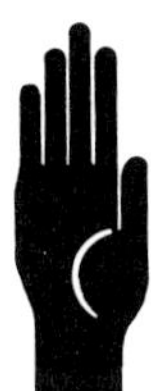

Satisfying Work

I go on working for the same reason that a hen goes on laying eggs.
—H.L. Mencken

My father taught me to work but not to love it. I never did like to work, and I don't deny it. I'd rather read, tell stories, crack jokes, talk, laugh—anything but work.
—Abraham Lincoln

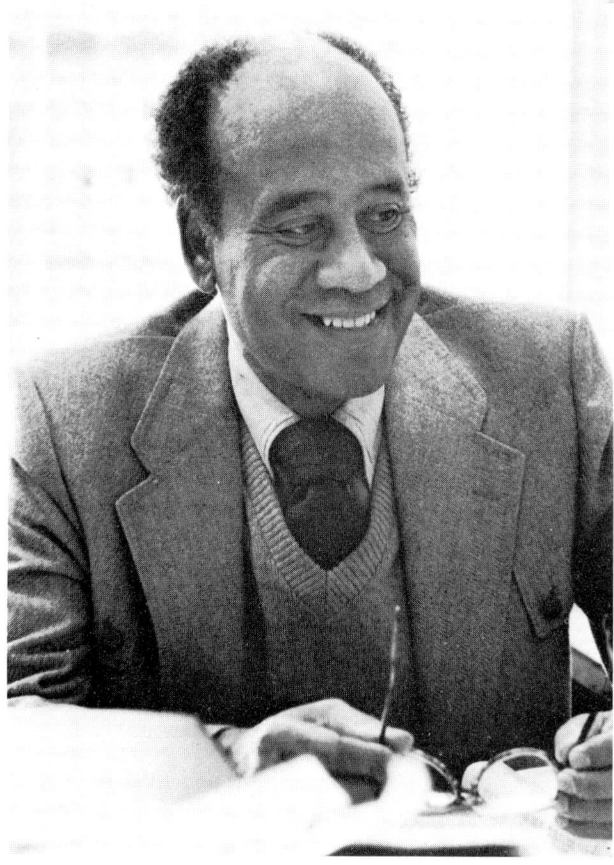

I don't mind being 60; the President of the country is over 70!
—Jim Davis

Many people 60 and over either have already retired from a long work life or will do so in the not too distant future. Some may be interested in continuing to work and earn money, either full-time or part-time, perhaps in a different kind of job. Others may be more interested in volunteering their time and experience, pursuing something that has meaning for them, keeping active and perhaps meeting new people.

For still other people, including those who have never worked outside their homes or haven't done so in many years, looking for rewarding work—paid or volunteer—may be something quite new.

Whatever category fits you best, looking for something satisfying to do may be one of the most important things at this stage in your life. This section of *60-PLUS* will give you information about a variety of places where you can find out both about paid work and about volunteer opportunities.

The following pages cover:

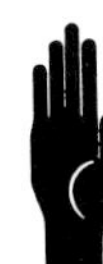

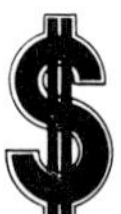

Paid employment

It *is* possible for people over 60 to find a good job. In every area of Massachusetts, there are employment services, state agencies, and other organizations that can help you find the kind of job that you want. You may have the chance to do on a part-time basis the same kind of work you once did full-time; or you may find a job doing what you always wanted to do but needed training for; or you may look for the first paid job of your life.

In addition to the services and programs listed below, you can get in touch with friends and former employers to find out about work opportunities.

Work and Social Security

You can earn up to $7,320* a year if you are over 65 without any reduction in your Social Security check. If you earn more than $7,320 by working, Social Security withholds $1 in benefits for each $2 earned over $7,320. This means that if you make $7,820 in 1985, Social Security will withhold $250 out of your yearly benefits.

If you know you will earn over $7,320 a year, you should report that to your local Social Security office as soon as possible. If you don't, all of the deductions will be withheld from the last few checks of the year which might leave you short on cash.

If you are over 70 years old, you will receive your full benefits each month no matter how much you earn.

*As of January 1985

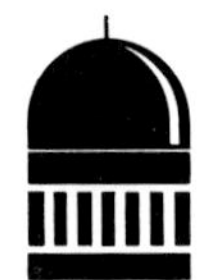

Two government-sponsored programs

A number of government-sponsored training and employment programs are available to help lower-income people enter or re-enter the labor force or get better jobs than they now have. Some of the jobs these programs lead to are in government or non-profit organizations, but many are in private business and industry. Typical kinds of help include: figuring out what kinds of work a person might do; training for new skills that might be needed on the job; and help in actually finding a job. Some programs are specifically for older workers.

JTPA (Job Training Partnership Act) Programs

These are job training and employment programs for people of all ages, that operate in 15 areas all around the state. The purpose of each program is to help people train for and find stable, long-term employment, primarily in private business and industry.

Generally, for you to be eligible for a JTPA program, your annual income *not counting* any Social Security benefits must be less than $5,250 (for a one-person household) or $7,050 (for a two-person household). Income limits are slightly different for some areas of the state; inquire when you call.

People who can participate include both those who are *not* working and those who *are* now working but want a new and better job.

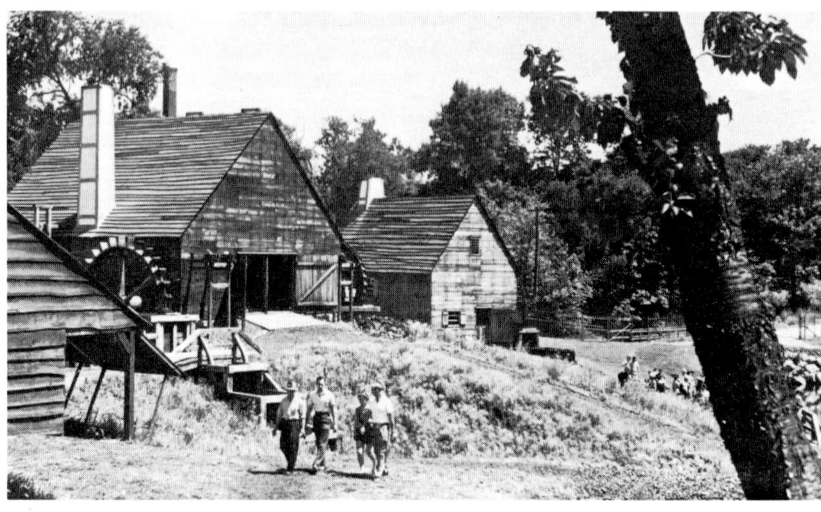

Saugus Ironworks
Saugus (617) 233-0050

The birthplace of the American steel industry can be seen as it appeared in 1650. National Historic Site. See No. 50, p.68.

To find out the telephone number for the JTPA office nearest you, call:

1-800-248-JOBS

Older Workers Programs. As part of JTPA, a number of programs specifically for people 55 and over have recently been set up on a pilot basis in eight areas of the state. Some programs provide training; all are interested in helping older workers find stable employment in suitable jobs.

Each area's program is different; the program near you might focus on jobs in retailing or home health care, word processing or computer data entry, clerical work or child care, or a wide variety of occupations. When you call your local JTPA office (see above), ask if there is an older workers' program and what it offers.

Senior Aides and other Senior Community Service Employment Programs

Have you ever heard of *Senior Aides?* It is one of several employment programs that offer people 55 and over the opportunity for paid work that is also of direct benefit to their community. As a participant you would work 20 hours a week for a private non-profit, non-sectarian community organization or for a government agency. If you were to need any training, it would be provided "on the job". The pay is at least minimum wage plus fringe benefits.

Jobs are available in many parts of Massachusetts and can range from tree planting and beautification to working in a senior center, social service agency, or library, to mention just a few examples. The jobs available will vary depending on the needs of the particular area and organization.

There are income limits to be eligible for one of these jobs: your annual income must be less than $6,225 (for a one-person household) or $8,400 (for a two-person household).* For the most part, these income limits *do* include your Social Security benefits.

There are five organizations that are responsible for these programs: the Executive Office of Elder Affairs; the National Urban League; Green Thumb; the American Association of Retired Persons; and the National Council of Senior Citizens.

To find out about opportunities in your area, and for more information about income requirements, write or call:

Executive Office of Elder Affairs
38 Chauncy Street
Boston, MA 02111
(617) **727-5948**
1-800-882-2003 (toll free)

Help in finding a job

Careers for Later Years/ Operation ABLE of Greater Boston

An affiliate of the Greater Boston Chamber of Commerce, Careers for Later Years is a non-profit organization dedicated to expanding employment opportunities for people 55 and over in the greater Boston area.

Through their Operation ABLE (Ability Based on Long Experience), they help employers to hire older workers and they help older job-seekers to find jobs.

ABLE accepts job listings from employers and makes those listings available to non-profit job-matching centers in the greater Boston area. ABLE also accepts inquiries from people looking for a job, and refers them to the center most likely to be helpful in matching the person with the right job. ABLE also gives listings of jobs and job-seekers to employment agencies.

If you are looking for a job in the greater Boston area, be sure to contact ABLE to see how they can help you:

ABLE Job Hotline
1-800-462-ABLE (toll free)
or (617) **338-0219**

An important source of help

All of the state's Home Care Corporations and Area Agencies on Aging offer help to older people looking for a job. In addition, there are several other nonprofit agencies that provide such assistance. Most will help you with your search at no

*As of August 1985

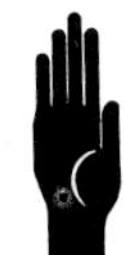

cost; if there is a fee they will tell you, and such a fee may be quite low and perhaps based on your ability to pay.

You will find the Home Care Corporation listed on pp. 54 - 55. The other organizations are listed below.

Boston (617) **725-3987**
Commission on Affairs of the Elderly

Boston (617) **266-3550**
Urban League of Eastern MA

Boston (617) **536-5651**
Women's Educational and Industrial Union

Brockton (617) **583-1833**
Old Colony Planning Council

Cambridge (617) **498-9039**
Prime Time

Hopedale (617) **473-3972**
Career Development Center

Newton (617) **552-7170**
Department of Human Services

Newton (617) **965-7940**
Jewish Vocational Service (nonsectarian)

Quincy (617) **471-5712**
Beechwood Community Life Center

Springfield (413) **781-7822,** ext. 3872
Springfield Tech. Community College

Worcester (617) **755-4388**
Age Center of Worcester

Worcester (617) **798-0191**
Catholic Charities (nonsectarian)

New toll-free number

Massachusetts state government, as part of its MASSJOBS program, has set up a central telephone number you can call—for help in finding a job, getting job training, locating employees for your business, and obtaining information on tax incentives for your business. You may call toll-free from anywhere in the state. When you call, you will be referred to the appropriate local office for the help you need.

1-800-248-JOBS

DES Job Matching Centers

Whether you are looking for full-time or part-time work, state government can help you—free of charge—through its Division of Employment Security (DES). DES maintains more than 35 offices throughout the state to help state residents of all ages to find jobs. These offices, known as Job Centers or Job Matching Centers, offer access to the largest list of job openings in Massachusetts and provide help both in using the job list and in contacting employers.

Since all offices have access to the same statewide computerized listing of job openings, you may use any of the offices and be assured that you will have the benefit of all the job information DES currently can make available to you.

Ask for the Senior Aide Some of the DES offices have a Senior Aide who works under the state Executive Office of Elder Affairs Senior Aide program. The Aide's job in the DES office is to help older workers find jobs. When you call or visit a DES office, be sure to ask if they have a Senior Aide there who is working on employment placement of older workers.

Greater Boston

Boston	Government Center **727-6320**
	Uphams Corner **282-6703**
Cambridge	**864-1950**
Framingham	**875-5238**
Malden	**322-8890**
Marlboro	**485-8711**
Norwood	**762-9450**
Waltham	**899-9340**
Woburn	**935-1396**

Northeastern

Gloucester	**283-4772**
Haverhill	**374-4753**
Lawrence	**682-5217**
Lowell	**458-4641**
Lynn	**593-5504**
Newburyport	**462-4494**
Salem	**745-1860**

Central

Fitchburg	343-6461
Gardner	632-5050
Milford	478-4300
Southbridge	765-5252
Webster	943-1240
Worcester	791-8551

Western

Chicopee	598-8371
Greenfield	774-4361
Holyoke	538-8271
North Adams	663-3748
Northampton	586-3116
Pittsfield	499-1793
Springfield	785-1231

Southeastern

Attleboro	222-1950
Brockton	586-8100
Fall River	678-8311
Hyannis	775-5800
New Bedford	999-2361
Plymouth	746-5910
Quincy	471-2750
Taunton	824-5835
Wareham	295-6170

If you are receiving welfare, the Division of Employment Security also offers intensive job development assistance through offices known as Employment Network Centers. To find out about the nearest Employment Network Center, call toll free **1-800-882-JOBS**.

ABCD (Action for Boston Community Development)
178 Tremont Street
Boston, MA 02111 **357-6000**

ABCD offers education and skills training in white-collar jobs and in culinary arts, and also acts as an employment referral service for workers in the Boston area who are looking for clerical, factory, and administrative and other positions. In addition, ABCD offers skill assessment and career planning for General Relief clients and will recommend employment and training options.

Other places to help you

Employment agencies can also be helpful; some, such as Mature Temps in Boston, are particularly interested in older workers. Your local **council on aging** pp. 81-83), your local **senior center,** and your area's **community college** are three other places which may be able to help you in your job search. And don't forget your **old employers**—you may be pleasantly surprised to find a welcome mat out for you, either from the same old managers or from new ones who have come in since you left. In each case, just make it clear that you are really looking for work, either on a full-time or part-time basis. There is a growing demand for mature, dependable workers, and you may meet with success much sooner than you think.

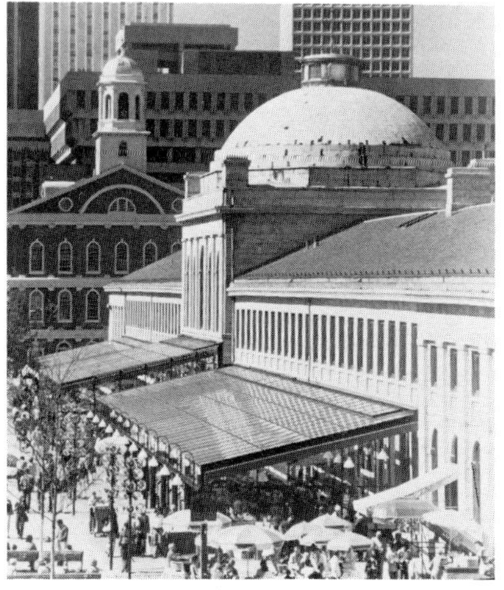

Quincy Market
Boston

One of the most popular places to visit in the country.

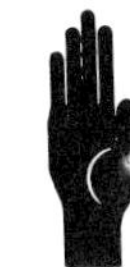

Do *you* know of a job?

Perhaps *you* can help an older person find a job—either because you have a job to offer or you know of a job in your company or organization. To list the job or get some help in filling it, here are some places to call:

Operation ABLE (Ability Based on Long Experience) of Greater Boston, Job Hotline: **1-800-462-ABLE** (toll free)

Mass. state government's central job number: **1-800-248-JOBS** (toll free)

Your local **council on aging, Home Care Corporation,** or **one of the organizations listed on p. 32.**

Starting your own business

You may also want to consider starting your own business. The Small Business Administration offers seminars at a nominal fee, free advice and all kinds of helpful publications. The District Office is in Boston, but there are SCORE volunteers (see p. 37) in all major cities in Massachusetts, usually in the Chamber of Commerce office. Look for the SCORE listing in your telephone directory, or write or call the District Office for more information:

Small Business Administration
150 Causeway Street
Boston, MA 02114
(617) **223-3237**

Sell what you make at home

If you make handcrafts at home and have an income under $7000 a year, one possible outlet for your work is Able Handcrafts of New England. This is a non-profit organization which is an outlet for handcrafts made in New England. Most of the craftspeople whose work they handle are over 60 years old. They have two stores, one in Boston near Quincy Market and another in Salem. They take on consignment handcrafts that have been approved by their quality review board (this review will take only a couple of days). They will help you set prices and tell you what items will sell. For example, "paintings just don't move," according to one Able staff member. For more information:

Able Handcrafts of New England
152 State Street
Boston, MA 02109
(617) **523-9096**

or

Able Handcrafts of New England
Salem Marketplace Derby Street
Salem, MA 01970
(617) **744-9633**

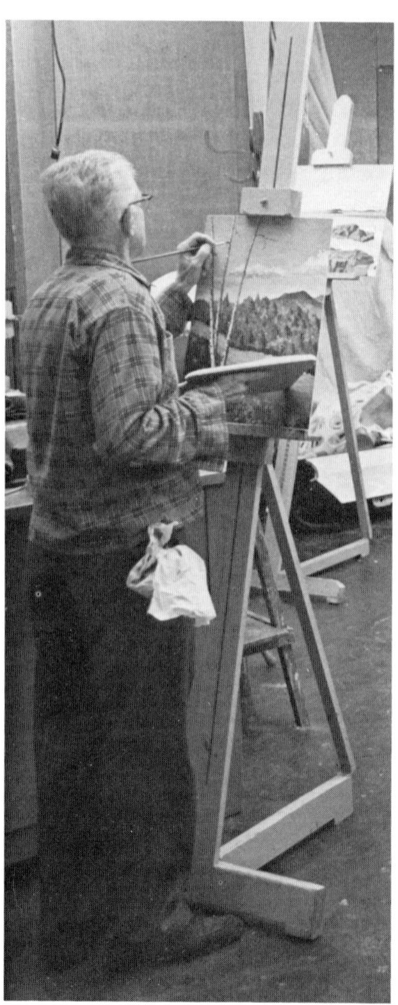

Taking a course. Art is one of many subjects offered by adult education centers and local museums. Call your council on aging for suggestions.

$ Volunteer jobs

No one is useless in this world who lightens the burden of another.
—Charles Dickens

You've learned a lot—share it! A complete list of volunteer jobs in Massachusetts would be hundreds or thousands of pages long. Volunteering is an invaluable service to others and to yourself. As you are busy helping, you are keeping your mind active and staying in touch with all kinds of people. It's never too late to make new friends. Why not put your experience to work?

Finding volunteer jobs

Boston area

Civic Center & Clearinghouse
14 Beacon Street
Boston, MA 02108
(617) **227-1762**

This organization has listings of volunteer positions in the Boston area and can also refer you to other organizations which have volunteer listings in other parts of the state. The Center also has a special program which offers counseling to women returning to work or getting a late start working.

Voluntary Action Center

United Way of Massachusetts Bay
87 Kilby Street
Boston, MA 02109
(617) **482-8370, ask for "VAC"**

The VAC helps people find places as volunteers in a variety of community projects and social service programs, at no charge.

Boston Aging Concerns

67 Newbury Street
Boston, MA 02116
(617) **266-2257**

An organization that can suggest many volunteer opportunities in the City of Boston.

Other areas

Information on volunteer jobs in other areas

Brockton area — **588-3460**
Old Colony Voluntary Action Center

Concord area — **369-1626**
Widening Horizons, Inc.

Framingham area — **875-5275**
Volunteers in Community Service

Leominster area — **534-3131**
United Way of North Central MA

Worcester area — **757-5631**
Voluntary Action Center

Your local hospital and library

One of the most rewarding places to volunteer is your local **hospital.** Your **visiting nurse association** or local **home care corporation** (see pp. 54-55) might also know of good volunteer opportunities in your area, and your local **library** is another good place to try.

Other suggestions

If you have a definite idea in mind, like working in an art gallery, try calling directly. Many places need reliable volunteers.

Or, you could become an active member of a group like your local council on aging that works to make life better for people over 60.

If you are interested in volunteer work, and enjoy a little exercise, you might offer your services as a fundraiser. A little legwork on your part can help find a cure for cancer or heart disease, or aid any number of good causes.

Volunteer listings in newspapers

Some newspapers, like the Boston Globe, provide listings of volunteer positions either every week or at specific times during the year.

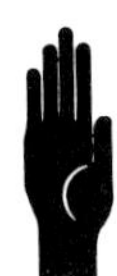

Some major volunteer programs

Listed below are programs that recruit older people for volunteer work. In some cases, a stipend (regular payment) or reimbursement for expenses is provided.

Elder Service Corps

Executive Office of Elder Affairs
38 Chauncy Street
Boston, MA 02111
Boston area: **727-5948**
Outside Boston area: **1-800-882-2003**

The Corps is a state-funded program which provides persons age 60 and over with a stipend to meet expenses they incur in doing volunteer work. Volunteers must enroll for a full year and work in various public and private non-profit human service agencies all across the state in programs related to the elderly. The monthly stipend is $110 for 18 hours of work a week or $220 for 37½ hours of work a week. Call to get the address and phone number of the program in your area.

Foster Grandparent Program

ACTION
441 Stuart Street
Boston, MA 02116
(617) **223-0590**

Low income people age 60 and over may work in this ACTION-funded program. A Foster Grandparent generally spends about four hours a day with a "special needs" child, five days a week, in a day-care center, a school, or a school for retarded children. Volunteers receive a tax-free stipend of $44.00 a week, reimbursement for transportation, a free meal daily, and on-the-job insurance. Foster Grandparent programs are now operating in Boston and in several other Massachusetts cities (see below). If you live elsewhere, call your local council on aging or ACTION to see if a program has been developed in your own community.

Boston (Suffolk County)	**357-6000, ext. 492**
Cambridge/eastern Middlesex County	**742-1326**
Fall River, Taunton, and surrounding towns	**679-0041**
Lowell and several surrounding towns	**459-0551**
New Bedford, Plymouth, and surrounding towns	**997-5425**
Springfield and many area communities	**739-7211**

ESCB—Executive Service Corps of Boston

Executive Service Corps of Boston
24 Federal Street
Boston, MA 02110
(617) **338-0213**

This volunteer program is for retired executives and professionals who want to help non-profit organizations solve management problems. It provides an opportunity to remain active, continue working with people, and take on the challenge of a new career in the non-profit world.

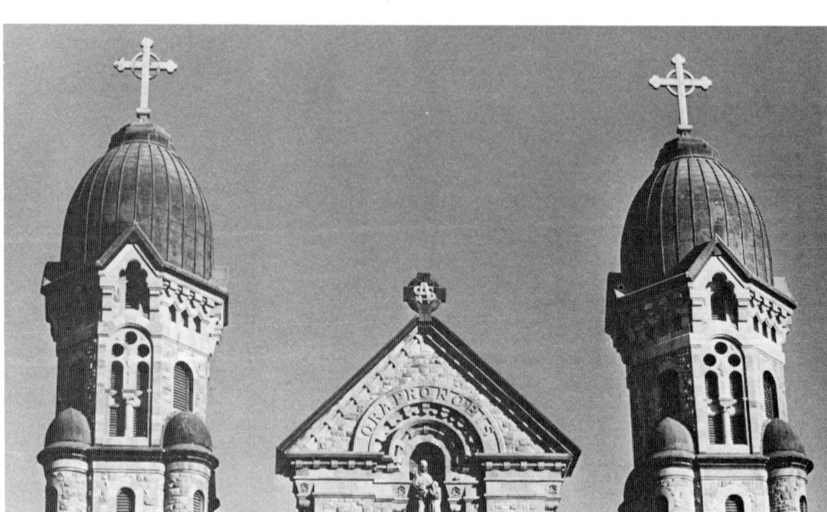

St. Anne's Church
Fall River

A landmark church with blue marble bell towers topped by Celtic crosses.

ESCB volunteers include former chief executive officers and professionals in such fields as accounting, law, finance, marketing, public relations, computers, and personnel management. Part of the non-profit Careers for Later Years, Inc., ESCB is patterned after the National Executive Service Corps in New York and is similar to services in more than 10 other cities.

Service Corps of Retired Executives (SCORE)

Small Business Administration
150 Causeway Street
Boston, MA 02114
(617) **223-3237**

SCORE volunteers are retired businessmen and women with management experience who help owners or managers—or *prospective* owners or managers—of small businesses and community organizations in need of management counseling. If your council on aging (see pp. 81-83) doesn't know of a local SCORE office, call or write the address above for information.

Veterans Hospital Volunteers

After receiving on-site orientation, volunteers help with such activities as letter writing, errands, reading, feeding patients, and recreation. Volunteers may also be asked to assist with admissions. As a volunteer, you are entitled to a free meal during your work hours.

To find out about volunteer opportunities, call the Chief of Voluntary Service at the nearest VA hospital.

Boston V.A. Medical Center	**232-9500**
West Roxbury V.A.	**323-7700**
Bedford V.A.	**275-7500**
Brockton V.A.	**583-4500**
Northampton V.A.	**584-4040**

SHINE

SHINE—Serving Health Information Needs of Elders—is a new volunteer program of the state's Executive Office of Elder Affairs. If you are a person with a strong interest or background in health insurance and benefits, and would like to work as a volunteer helping older people understand how to meet their needs for adequate health insurance, contact your local council on aging (pp. 81-83) or:

Executive Office of Elder Affairs
38 Chauncy Street
Boston, MA 02111
(617) **727-4092**
1-800-882-2003 (toll free)

Peace Corps

Room 1304
150 Causeway Street
Boston, MA 02114
(617) **223-7366**

The Peace Corps actively recruits older people to serve a minimum of two years as overseas volunteers in developing countries. While in training and during service, volunteers receive a generous monthly allowance for food, travel, rent, and all medical needs. After they come back, each is paid a "readjustment allowance" of over $4,000 in a lump sum.

VISTA

441 Stuart Street, 9th floor
Boston, MA 02116
(617) **223-0590**

VISTA (Volunteers in Service to America) is the domestic version of the Peace Corps. VISTA volunteers receive a limited subsistence allowance which will not affect their Social Security benefits. The "readjustment allowance" is $900 after one year of volunteer work. You may volunteer to work either in your own community or in another part of the country.

Retired Senior Volunteer Program (RSVP)

ACTION
441 Stuart Street
Boston, MA 02116
(617) **223-0590**

R.S.V.P. is sponsored by ACTION—the federal funding agency—to give people 60 and over the opportunity to contribute their time, experience, knowledge and interest to others in their own community. There are R.S.V.P. programs in hospitals, libraries, courts, museums,

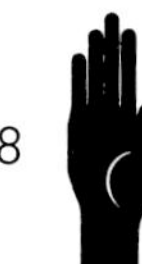

senior centers, day care centers, schools, and many other places. Volunteers may be reimbursed, upon request, for meals, transportation, and have their insurance supplemented. Call or write the address above for more information about your area.

School Volunteers

Boston. School Volunteers for Boston, a private non-profit agency, recruits and trains volunteers to work in Boston public schools. Volunteers may do tutoring, assist in libraries and classrooms, provide special information on careers or historical events, act as role models, and form loving friendships with children. A flexible schedule is available to volunteers. If you are over 55, you will be reimbursed for travel.

School Volunteers for Boston, Inc.
25 West Street
Boston, MA 02111
(617) **451-6145**

Other cities. There is a similar program in most larger cities. Ask your local Board of Education or School Department if your community has such a program, or call the number listed above.

Senior Companion Program

ACTION
441 Stuart Street
Boston, MA 02116
(617) **223-0590**

Low income people age 60 and over and in good health are eligible to serve as volunteers, visiting older people in their homes to provide them with companionship. A Senior Companion gets a tax-free stipend, reimbursement for transportation, a free meal, and supplementary insurance. Five current programs are listed below. If you live elsewhere, call ACTION or your local Home Care Corporation (see pp. 54-55) to find out if a program has been developed in your own community.

Fitchburg/Gardner	**345-7312**
Lowell area	**459-0551**
Milford	**473-4800**
Southbridge	**764-2501**
Worcester area	**755-4388**

MATCH-UP

Boston Aging Concerns
67 Newbury Street
Boston, MA 02116
(617) **266-2257**

Friendship, companionship, support—if these are what you would like to provide as a volunteer, there are many opportunities for you to help another person in the City of Boston. Through its MATCH-UP program, Boston Aging Concerns will pair you with someone whom you can visit, talk with, help with such things as reading and letter writing, escort on errands, and whose friendship *you* will enjoy.

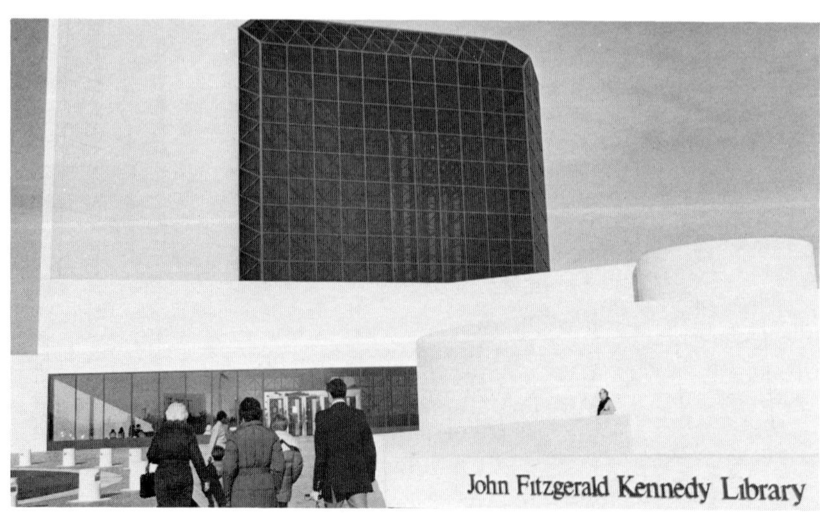

John Fitzgerald Kennedy Library Museum
Dorchester (617) 929-4523

The spectacular Presidential Library at Columbia Point was built with funds donated by people from all over the world. See No. 38, p.67.

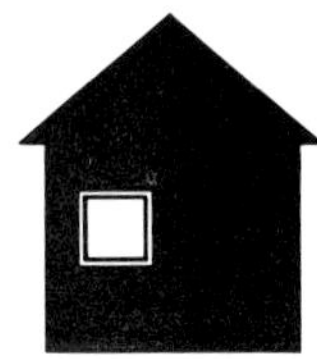

Your Home

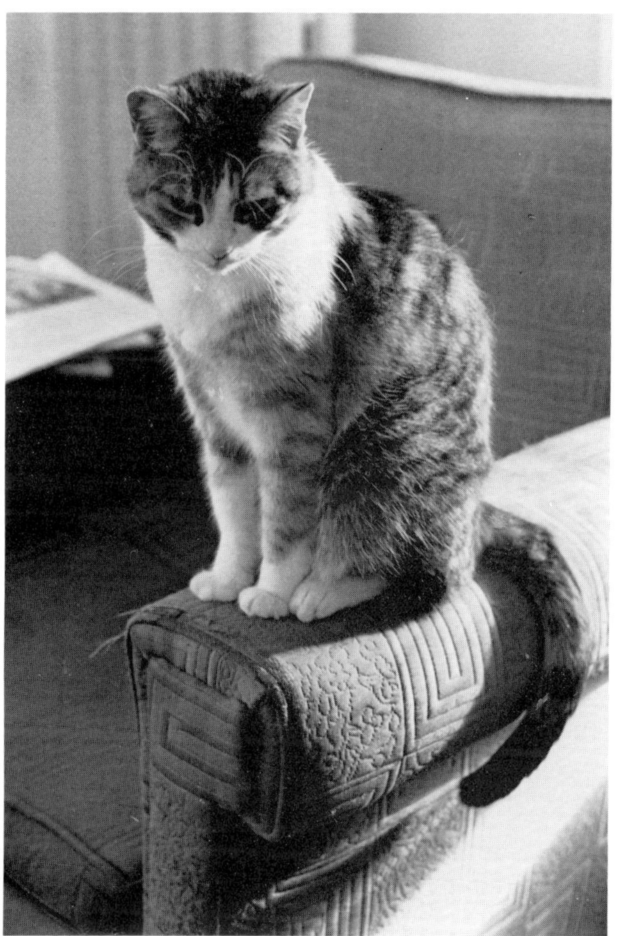

It takes a heap o' livin' in a house
t' make it a home. . .
—Edgar Albert Guest

At some point you may want to move—to an apartment; from a big apartment to a smaller one; from a place where you live alone to a home you share with someone else; or to a place where others will help care for you.

Or you may want to stay right where you are, but make some changes or get someone to share or help.

Figuring out the best thing to do about your housing arrangements is one of the most important decisions for you to make. To make the right choice—especially if you are thinking of moving—talk it over with friends, family, and other people you trust and who know you. But once you have their advice and opinions, make sure *you* feel the decision is the right one.

The next few pages will give you an idea of what your choices are should you decide to stay or to move.

This section covers:

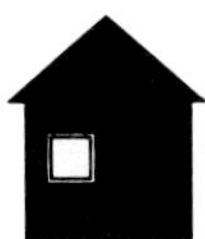

Staying where you are

For any number of reasons, staying where you are, rather than moving, may be the right housing choice for you. Even so, there may be some important changes and improvements that can make life happier, more comfortable, and more affordable.

Someone to share your home with you

For companionship or to reduce your expenses, you may want to have someone share your home with you. It could be a relative, a friend, or someone new.

If you don't already know someone who might share your home with you, ask your local council on aging (pp. 81-83), your Home Care Corporation (pp. 54-55), your clergyman, or look in your local paper for someone advertising for a place to live. There may also be a "home sharing" program in your area, which can put you in touch with people looking for such an arrangement; contact your council on aging or Home Care Corporation.

If you don't want to share your entire home, you might rent a room or two, perhaps with kitchen privileges. Local regulations usually permit this, but check with your town or city hall to make sure.

Another possibility is to create an **"accessory apartment"** by setting aside part of your house, or the space over your garage, as a separate rental unit. This may mean you need to have an additional outside entrance constructed or make other structural changes. If your house or garage lends itself to this, you will need to get permits from the appropriate authorities in your city or town government. Not all communities allow accessory apartments; call your town or city hall to find out *before* you do any construction or rent out such an apartment.

Mail order safety and comfort

There are many things on the market to make life safer and more comfortable at home. Few stores carry a wide selection, however. Shopping by mail can be an easier way to get what you need.

These two unusual catalogs contain many items that may be of interest—from bathroom comfort and safety products, to gardening tools, to scissors and other things for people with arthritis, and many household, clothing, sickroom and personal care items. Both catalogs include some ingenious and useful things you probably didn't know even existed. While some things may not suit your lifestyle or budget, many others may meet a real need for you or someone you know.

The Capability Collection Catalog
$2.50 (refundable with minimum $30.00 purchase) from:
Ways and Means™
28001 Citrin Drive
Romulus, MI 48174
1-800-654-2345 toll free

Comfortably Yours® Catalog
$2.00 from:
Aids for Easier Living
52 West Hunter Avenue
Maywood, NJ 07607

Some of the things in the *Capability Collection Catalog* are also available in "centers" in retail stores; you can call to inquire about exact store locations. You may also be interested in the Sears *Home Health Catalog* (see p. 59).

Someone to help you

Having someone come in to help you from time to time may be the real key to living comfortably at home. Your area's Home Care Corporation (pp. 54-55) can tell you about the kinds of home care services available to you. Your local Visiting Nurse Association is another important source of help and information about home care. Finally, you may be able to exchange room and board for some help on a regular basis—this might be an ideal non-cash arrangement for someone you let share your home with you.

Making your home safer and more livable

There are many ways to make your home a better place to live—safer, more comfortable, easier to manage. While this can benefit anyone, it can be of prime importance for a person who has a disability—hearing, seeing, walking, etc. Incidentally, contrary to what many people believe, the great majority of people over 60 do *not* have a disability.

Improvements for your home can range from better lighting and rearranging where you store things, to handrails, ramps, and other "adaptations" that require some construction or special equipment.

One organization that specializes in helping people determine what improvements to make is the Adaptive Environments Center in Boston. They have free publications, a reference library, and a list of experienced contractors; they also offer a three-hour "home audit" (fee $200) that will result in specific recommendations for your home.

Adaptive Environments Center
Mass. College of Art
621 Huntington Avenue
Boston, MA 02115
(617) **739-0088**

You may be able to get some financial assistance for special improvements from your area's Home Care Corporation (see pp. 54-55) or from some other organization (ask the Adaptive Environments Center, above, if they know of other sources of loans or grants).

Moving somewhere new

Moving is a *major* decision. It may turn out to be just the right thing for you to do, but it can also be a very unsettling change and possibly even a real mistake. Because where you live is not just a house or an apartment—it's the friends and family, the neighborhood, the stores, the places to work and worship, all the things nearby, as well as the associations and memories of perhaps many years of living in that place. So, no matter where you're considering moving, give it a lot of thought.

Test out a distant move. If you are thinking of moving to a totally new environment, perhaps far away, try it *before* you make the move. Visit with a friend there, or rent a place for a short time. After actually staying there, you may find that in reality the new place is not what you pictured in your mind or saw in a brochure. *Or* you may conclude it's a nice place for a vacation but not somewhere to move on a permanent basis.

Don't move too soon. Be very careful not to make a permanent move too soon after the death of your spouse or another loved one. The familiar surroundings that seem so empty at first may be a source of comfort and of happy memories after the initial shock has passed. Also, since it's such a traumatic time, it may be especially hard to make a really good decision, even if moving *is* the right thing to do. Take your time.

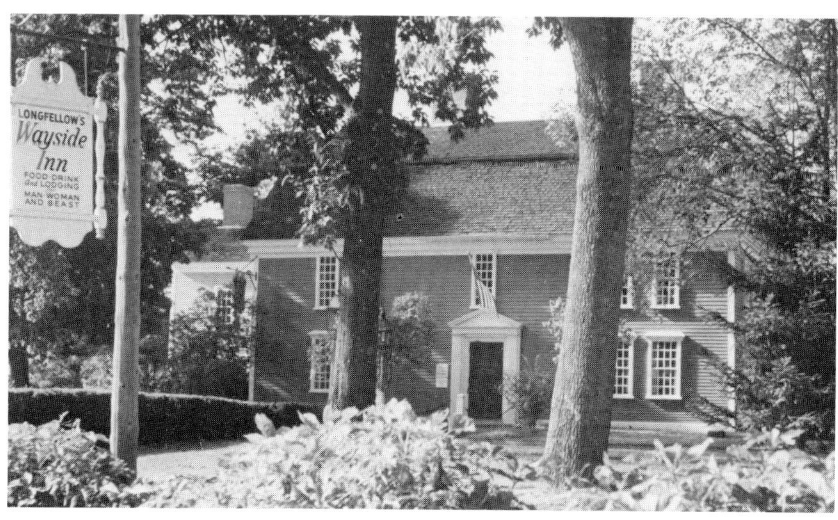

Wayside Inn
Sudbury

Made famous by Longfellow's "Tales of a Wayside Inn," the inn has been visited by many famous Americans, including George Washington.

Enjoying Massachusetts

Historic homes

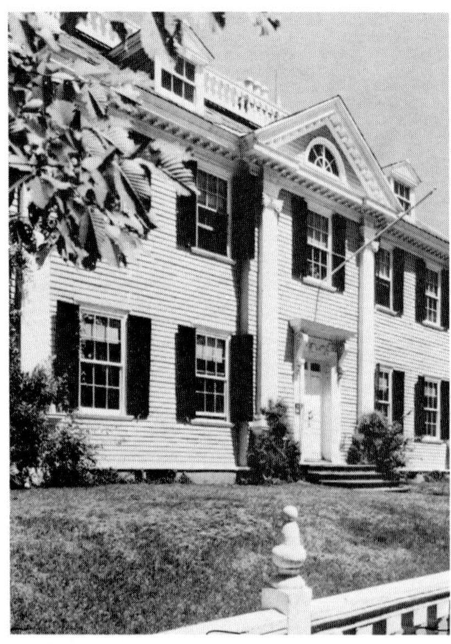

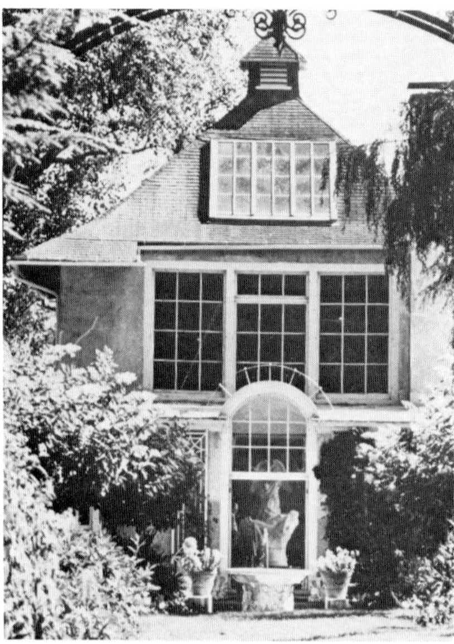

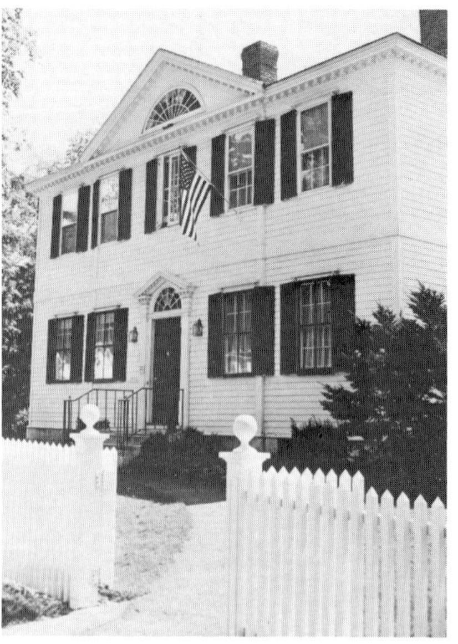

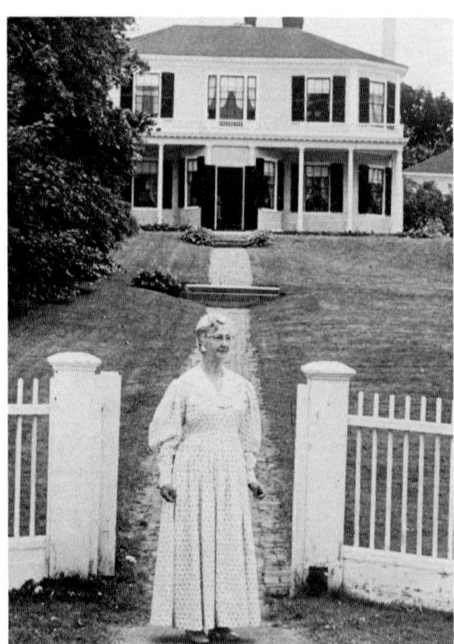

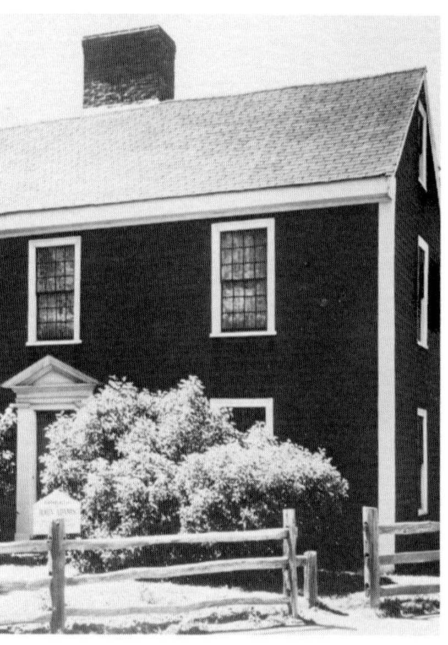

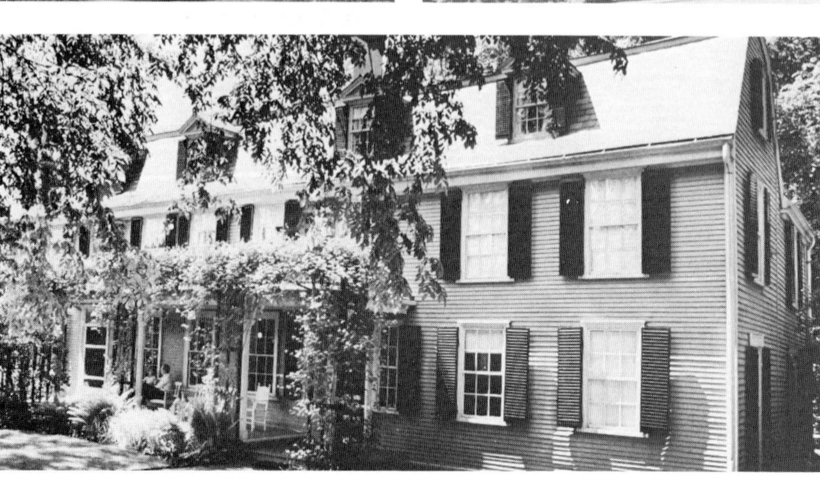

Left to right from top:

Longfellow National Historic Site
Cambridge (617) 876-4491
House where Henry Wadsworth Longfellow wrote many of his best known poems. See No. 34, p.67.

Chesterwood
Stockbridge (413) 298-3579
Take a tour of sculptor Daniel Chester French's studio, residence, Barn Sculpture Gallery and a nature trail. See No. 72, p.69.

Norman Rockwell Museum
Stockbridge (413) 298-3822
An 18th century landmark with Norman Rockwell paintings on display. See No. 73, p.69.

The Antiquarian House
Plymouth
Built in 1809, the Antiquarian House is furnished as a 19th century merchant's home. See No. 14, p.65.

John Adams Birthplace
Quincy (617) 773-1177
Birthplace of the second President of the United States. See No. 40, p.67.

Adams National Historic Site
Quincy (617) 773-1177
Built in 1731, the Adams home and grounds reflect the tastes of the four generations of the Adams family who made it their home.

Finding a place

If you decide to move outside of Massachusetts, there are many books in your library and in bookstores that can give you insights into different areas. If you are thinking of moving within Massachusetts, you may want to consider the following.

Special housing for people who want to live on their own

There is housing available in many cities and towns that has been specially designed to make it comfortable and convenient for older people to live in. These special design features may include higher electric outlets so you don't have to lean over so far to plug in an appliance, fewer stairs or perhaps even an elevator, an emergency alarm system or intercom, kitchen cabinets at just the right height, or special bathroom fixtures such as handrails to help you climb in and out of the tub. While the special features vary from one place to another, all of this housing is limited to people over a certain age; in some cases, however, handicapped people of all ages are eligible, too.

Private developers have built special rental apartments or condominiums like this in many parts of the state. Although there aren't any huge retirement communities (like Sun City, Arizona) in Massachusetts, there are many smaller complexes. Sales or rentals are limited to people 55 and over whose children, if living with them, are 16 and over. Check with a real estate agent to find out about this kind of housing in the community where you want to live.

Nonprofit real estate developers—perhaps a community organization or a religious group—have also built special housing for older people. These are almost always rental units, and the rent charged is based on people's ability to pay.

Usually, if you are a *single* person, you must be over 62 to qualify; but there are no age limits for a disabled or handicapped person or for a husband or wife of someone who qualifies. You pay approximately one quarter of your income in rent. There are overall income limits, and your assets are also taken into account.

Check with town or city Housing Authorities in your area to see if this kind of housing is available for you. Check with your council on aging if your town doesn't have a Housing Authority. This kind of housing is in short supply, and the waiting list may be long.

Public housing for older people has been built in communities throughout Massachusetts. It is frequently the least expensive housing choice available. This kind of housing is usually limited to people 65 and over. The income qualifications may vary from community to community. You may apply for public housing in communities other than the one in which you now live.

Many public housing complexes have large rooms for special activities and entertainment, and some have apartments specially designed for people in wheelchairs. Interesting new examples of public housing for older people include the converted mill buildings in Lowell and Stoughton and the former school buildings in Peabody and Norwood. Since you will probably have to wait anywhere from a month to more than a year for an apartment, it is important to apply *before* you are ready to move.

Call the Housing Authorities in your area for more information.

A helpful publication

In April 1984, state government published a helpful guide entitled, "How to Obtain Housing Assistance in Massachusetts: A Handbook of Housing Resources", which includes explanations of housing programs and listings of local housing agencies throughout the Commonwealth. A large section is devoted to a directory of privately owned subsidized housing developments in many cities and towns. For a free copy, write or call:

Executive Office of Communities and Development
100 Cambridge Street, 14th floor
Boston, MA 02202
(617) **727-7130**

Some special living arrangements

Shared living arrangements. There are several kinds of shared living arrangements available in Massachusetts. For instance **congregate housing** is housing in which older people have their own rooms but share some common rooms and cooking facilities. These residences do not usually provide health care, and the people who live in them make all their own decisions about health care and activities. There are now about 14 state-funded congregate housing developments in various cities and towns, as well as some private and some federally funded ones. Over the next few years nearly 50 additional state-funded developments will be built.

In most shared housing, people do their own cooking, cleaning, and shopping. But other kinds of services are sometimes offered, like: more janitorial support than in conventional apartment buildings; recreational counselors; and social workers.

The cost of living in shared housing varies, and so do the age limits. Some residences are state supported and are for low income people; for others you would need to have an annual income of more than $10,000.

If you are interested in a shared living arrangement, call the Housing Authority in your city or town or your council on aging (see pp. 81-83) for more information.

"Shared Living: What Is It? Would I Like It?", and "Shared Living: An Individual Planning Guide" are two brochures that should be helpful to anyone who wants to explore this type of living arrangement. Each is $2.00, for postage and handling, from:

ABCD, Inc.
Community Services Department
178 Tremont Street
Boston, MA 02111

Information about congregate housing, and about existing and new developments near you, is available from:

Congregate Housing Specialist
Executive Office of Elder Affairs
38 Chauncy Street
Boston, MA 02111
(617) **727-0690**

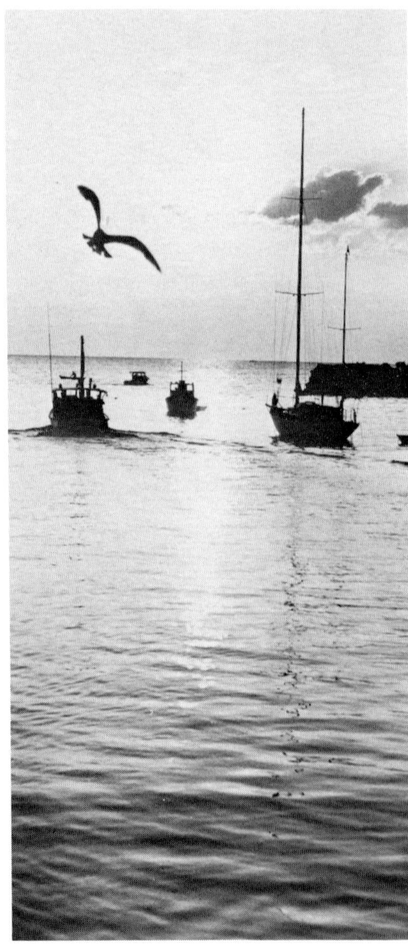

Rockport Harbor entrance
Rockport is one of the oldest artist colonies in Massachusetts.

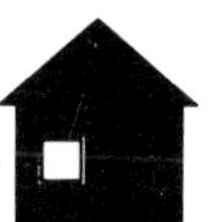

"Lifecare" housing complexes, still uncommon in Massachusetts, offer a blend of housing and services—housekeeping, meals, laundry, social activities, personal and health care. Usually privately owned, they provide a long-term, eviction-free, and care-free living situation. Residents "buy in" with a substantial membership fee which may be returned in whole or in part whenever a member gives up the apartment. Massachusetts communities where lifecare complexes are located include: Bedford, Brockton, and Needham. Quite popular in other parts of the country, lifecare housing is likely to increase in Massachusetts in the coming years.

Adult foster care. If an older person can no longer live safely alone at home, one possibility may be to move into someone else's home where not only shelter but also some care will be provided. This is a housing/care alternative for people who prefer to live in a family setting in a home, rather than in an institution, but do *not* require round-the-clock care.

Adult foster care is a program that is open to all, regardless of income, and costs about $950 a month.* There are now at least 12 adult foster care programs around the state, that help match people to suitable homes and provide ongoing health care. For the program in your area, call your area's Home Care Corporation (pp. 54-55).

Homes for retired people or "rest homes" are an alternative if you don't want to fix your own meals or if you find it hard to get out to see people. Most rest homes provide meals, activities, staff nurses, and transportation to shopping areas for residents. They are planned with the needs of older people in mind.

If you are thinking about moving into a rest home, plan ahead. There is often a long wait. Make appointments at several rest homes and bring a list of questions, including these:

- What health care is available?
- What is the waiting time before moving in?
- How many staff members and how many residents are there?
- What transportation and recreational services are provided?

Ask if you can stay for a meal and talk to people who live there.

To find out about rest homes in your area, call your council on aging (see pp. 81-83).

*As of July 1985

Nursing or convalescent homes provide all the health care that can be handled outside a hospital. Meals and laundry are also provided. There is a wide range of cost and quality in nursing homes, so choose carefully. The Nursing Home Ombudsman (617-**727-7273**) will tell you what nursing homes there are in your area but will not recommend any. Before selecting a nursing home, you should really read up on the things to look for and ask about. But here are some basic pointers:

- Ask the nursing home for recommendations;
- Visit several;
- Ask questions;
- Ask the local council on aging (see pp. 81-83) what they know about different nursing homes.

It doesn't take long to get the "feel" of a place, but there are certain things to look for. Tell-tale signs of a place to stay *away* from include: lack of privacy; most people being in bed rather than dressed, up and about; staff who don't know people's names; very restricted visiting hours; poor food; or, few personal possessions in people's rooms.

Helpful publications

"A Guide to Nursing and Rest Homes in Massachusetts" explains levels of care and other essentials, and provides information about each of the nursing and rest homes licensed by the state's Department of Public Health. To order a copy, send a check for $7.19 (includes postage) made out to the organization which publishes the guide:

Women's Educational and Industrial Union
Social Services Department
356 Boylston Street
Boston, MA 02116

"A Consumers Guide to: Selecting a Nursing Home" is an introductory booklet which also lists local "ombudsman" organizations throughout the state. A free copy may be obtained from:

Executive Office of Elder Affairs
Nursing Home Ombudsman Division
38 Chauncy Street
Boston, MA 02111
(617) **727-7273**

If you have a complaint against a nursing home, see page 76.

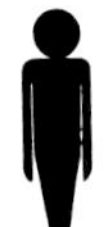

If you own a house

Your house may be your most valuable personal asset. If you decide to sell it, don't let any personal crisis prevent you from getting its full value. **Dont' sell it without expert advice.** The price of houses in most parts of Massachusetts has gone up dramatically. Even if you knew what your house was worth two years ago, values have changed so much since then that you owe it to yourself to make sure you know its value *today*. And your property tax assessment may *not* be a good clue to what your house is worth.

The best way to find out the current value of your house is to have it appraised by a knowledgeable local real estate professional. Your bank may be able to recommend one. If you decide to sell the house, it may also be better to employ a professional than to sell it yourself. Real estate agents probably have better access to buyers and can be enormously helpful in negotiating the best price. Yes, they do take a commission on the sale, but the higher the sale price the bigger their commission will be. So they have an interest in getting the most they can for your house.

Some towns and cities offer technical or financial assistance to help you **repair or rehabilitate your home**. If you live in a town of fewer than 10,000 people, check with the nearest Farmers Home Administration office. It is an agency of the U.S. government. They offer both low interest loans for low income people of all ages and direct grants to low income people over 62 to remove safety or health hazards from their homes. The maximum loan or grant you can get from the Farmers Home Administration is $5,000.* Apply at the Farmers Home Administration office near you. The offices are located in:

Amherst 253-3471
Bourne 759-2136
Gardner 632-1864
Hadley 584-7992
Holden 829-6626
Littleton 486-8917
Pittsfield 443-9624
Raynham 822-7141

Some cities and towns have special programs to help people repair or improve their homes. These programs vary from year to year and from city to city.

One such program, for elderly Boston homeowners, can make minor repairs needed in your home, help you obtain a tenant for an underused or vacant rental unit you may have, and help provide maintenance services. There is a small annual fee. Call to see if you are eligible for help.

Housing Assistance Program for Elderly Homeowners
Ecumenical Social Action Committee
20 South Street
Jamaica Plain, MA 02130
(617) **524-4820**

*As of April 1985

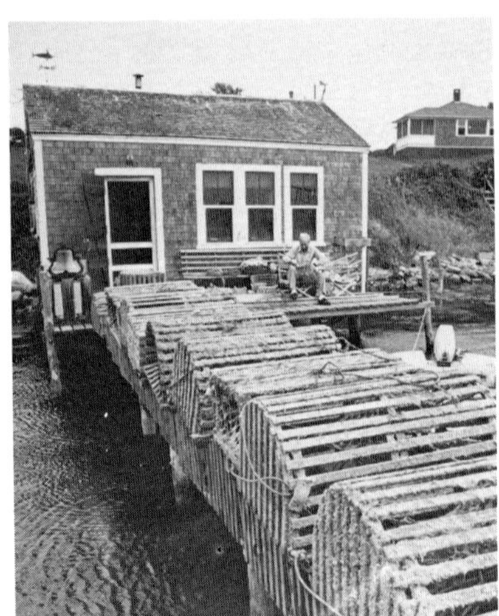

◂ **Lobster Pots**
Martha's Vineyard

Lobster fisherman working on his traps.

Rooster weathervane ▸
Chatham

Roosters, whalers and sailing ships are common weathervane motifs along the Massachusetts seacoast.

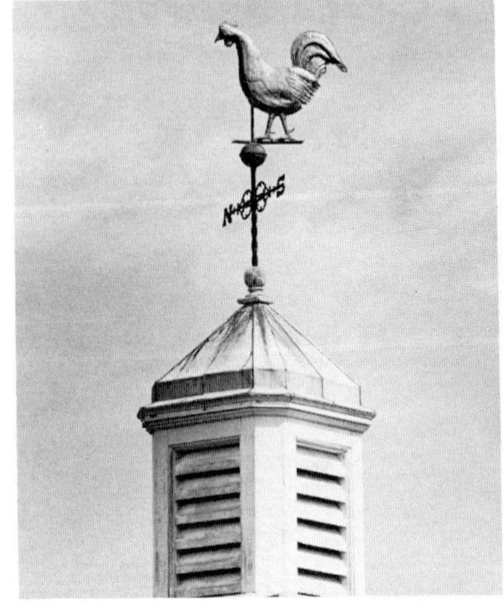

Sometimes only a few neighborhoods are eligible for special home repair programs. To find out if there is such a program in your community and whether or not you are eligible, call your town or city hall and ask for the Redevelopment Authority, community economic development corporation, or community development agency.

Freeing up the equity in your home. Your home may be your most valuable financial asset. In order to meet some cash needs, you may want to "tap into" the capital—the equity—in your home.

Problem: how to free up that capital without selling your home and moving. One answer is **home equity conversion**. By using a *reverse mortgage* from a bank, a *sale-leaseback* arrangement, or some other method, it may be possible to have some of the equity in cash to use now and still continue to live in your house.

Home equity conversion is just starting to be used by older people in Massachusetts, and only a few banks are currently originating reverse mortgage loans. For more information on how home equity conversion works, call or write one of the following:

Senior Home Equity Project
ABCD
178 Tremont Street
Boston, MA 02111
(617) **357-6000**, Ext. 289

Executive Office of Elder Affairs
Housing Policy Analyst
38 Chauncy Street
Boston, MA 02111
(617) **727-0690**

Other assistance. See page 17 about help from the government to pay your **heating bill**. See pages 20-22 about property **tax deferments** and the **exclusion of gain** on the sale of your house. See pp. 54-55 for information on the **Home Care** Corporation that can help you stay in your present home as long as possible.

$ Your rights as a tenant

What are your rights as a tenant in Massachusetts? The different cities and towns in the state make their own laws about some issues such as rent control and condominium conversions, but most rights you have as a tenant are enforceable in all cities and towns under Massachusetts state laws.

Evictions and rent increases

Whether or not you have a lease, state law protects you against abrupt eviction. You have **time** after receiving an eviction notice, and you *may* not have to lose your home at all. The eviction notice must be **in writing** and in the proper form. Furthermore, remember that **a landlord cannot evict you; only a judge** can do that, and *after* you have had an opportunity for a court hearing. In many situations, you may have from six months to a year to find a new place to live. **Do not panic** if you receive a telephone call or even a written notice from your landlord that you are about to be evicted. But *do* get some legal advice (see p. 49).

As for rent increases, **if you have no lease** (a "tenant-at-will"), you *do* have some protection. First, the landlord must notify you **in writing** that the old rent will end, and there must be a full rental period (say, you have been paying weekly or monthly) between when you receive the notice and when the new rent would start. Secondly, the landlord must offer you the right to stay in your home at the new and higher rent. If you choose not to pay the new rent, be sure to continue to pay the old rent on time. Then, if the landlord wants you evicted for not accepting the new rent, the landlord must take you to court. Remember, **only a judge** can order an eviction.

If you have a lease, your rent level is protected by that lease until it ends. If your lease includes an option to renew, you may be protected well beyond—*if* you properly exercise your option (usually well before the lease ends).

If you are to be evicted for not accepting a rent increase, this is called a "no fault" eviction. Massachusetts law protects tenants who are 60 and over, or who are handicapped, by allowing the judge to give the tenant **up to one full year** to find another place to live. The tenant **must ask** the judge for that time, however.

In Boston and other communities where there is rent control there is further protection for tenants. And there may be circumstances where a tenant cannot be evicted at all.

To be sure you know your rights in a specific situation, you should be sure to get some legal advice (see p. 49) as soon as you have been notified of a possible eviction or rent increase. In addition, you may want to contact the Mass. Tenants Organization tion (see phone number on p. 49) to inquire about printed information on tenants' rights.

Problems with the condition of your home

You also have certain rights according to state law to protect you when a landlord does not provide adequate facilities or maintenance. For instance, if you have cockroaches, broken plumbing, no heat or hot water, or other problems, those may be violations of the State Sanitary Code. For a **Housing Code Checklist** of all the conditions that are violations of the State Sanitary Code, send $1.00 to:

Mass. Tenants Organization
14 Beacon Street
Boston, MA 02108

The checklist is available in English, Spanish or French. There is also a free folder, called *Safe and Sanitary Housing,* which you can get from the Mass. Secretary of State's office:

Citizen Information Service
One Ashburton Place
Boston, MA 02108
(617) **727-7030**
1-800-392-6090 (toll free)

Your first step must be to ask the landlord to take care of the problem. Put your complaint in writing and keep a copy for yourself. If you live in an apartment house, ask the other tenants in your building if they have complaints about the condition of their apartments. If they do and you can complain together, your are likely to be more effective.

If your landlord doesn't take care of the problem after a reasonable period of time, you can file a complaint. Every city or town has a housing inspector or health inspector whose job is to investigate complaints about violations of the State Sanitary Code. The name of the department these inspectors work in changes from place to place. For example, in Boston, it's called the Housing Inspection Division; in Brockton, the Housing Code Division; in Fall River, the Sanitary Code Department.

Call your town or city hall and ask for the right phone number to report a violation of the State Sanitary Code. Make an appointment with the housing inspector to come inspect your apartment.

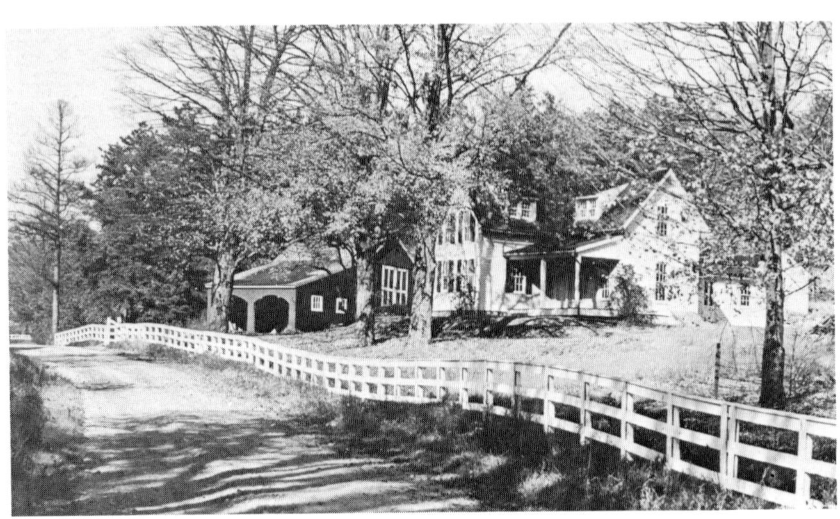

Autumn in Massachusetts

You can take a train to see beautiful fall foliage. See p.64 for more information.

Make sure you take the name of the inspector for future reference. Sometimes landlords turn up at the same time as the inspector. Don't let that bother you. Point out all the problems you have with the condition of your apartment and make sure you haven't cleaned up all of your best evidence, like dead cockroaches or rat droppings. If the inspector decides that the problems in your apartment are hazardous, strong measures will be taken to make your landlord clear up the violations.

If an inspector certifies that your complaint is serious and your landlord hasn't begun to make repairs within a certain number of days, there are several legal steps you could take. These steps include withholding the rent and paying for the repairs yourself. Before you take action on your own, check with a lawyer.

Getting legal advice

Proper legal advice is very important in housing matters. See p. 52 for how to find a lawyer. You can also get information and advice on your housing rights from:

Mass. Tenants Organization (a membership organization—they'll ask you to join: $5 if you are on a fixed income)
(617) **367-6260**

Greater Boston Elderly Legal Services
(617) **536-0400.** See p. 52 for information.

Legal Advocacy and Research Center
(617) **542-8787**

A landlord may not retaliate

Massachusetts law protects you if your landlord retaliates against you for making a complaint. For example, your landlord may not shut off your electricity.

If you live in public housing

If you do not have a private landlord but live in *public* housing, talk with your Housing Authority staff and with any tenants' committee or group that may exist to cope with problems. This organization is also an excellent source of information and support:

Mass. Union of Public Housing Tenants
(617) **262-0348**

Other assistance

As a tenant you may also be interested in the **fuel assistance** program that can pay part of your heating bill (see p. 17) or the **Home Care** Corporations that will help you to stay in your present home as long as possible (see pp. 54-55). And did you know that your landlord owes you **5% interest on your security deposit** every year on the anniversary of your lease or your first rent payment?

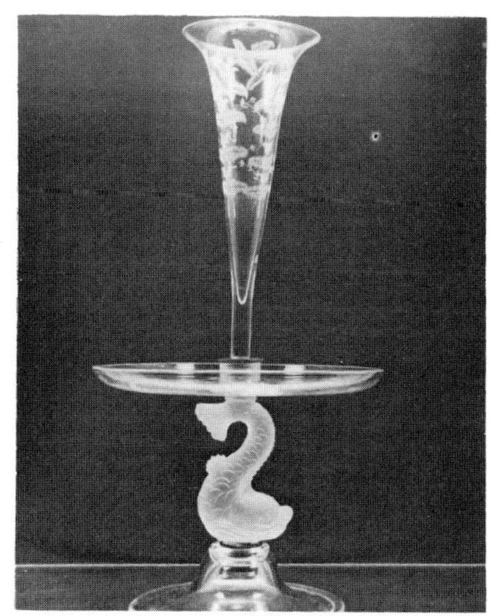

Sandwich Glass Museum
Sandwich (617) 888-0251

A piece from the collection of rare Sandwich Glass, made from 1825 to 1888 in the Boston and Sandwich Glass Company factory. See No. 5, p.65.

Protection from utility cutoff

All the utility companies in Massachusetts—gas companies, electric companies and the telephone company—have made a special provision for homes in which *all* adult residents are 65 years old or older. A public utility *cannot discontinue service* without the written approval of the Massachusetts Department of Public Utilities.

To protect yourself against possible service cutoffs, all you need to do is to call the business office of your telephone company or the customer division of your electric or gas utility and ask for the "Age 65 or over Notification Card." These cards also come periodically with your bill. Once you have filled out the card and sent it in, you won't need to do it again and your service will be protected permanently against routine cutoff.

The notification card also gives you a chance to ask that notices of past due bills for your account be sent to a friend, relative or neighbor—anyone you choose. Then if you are sick or away from home, this person will be able to check with you or contact the utility on your behalf. This person will *never* be required to pay the bill.

If you are *under* 65 and have a financial hardship that prevents you from paying your utility bill, you are protected from your electricity being shut off if: you or someone living in your home is seriously ill; or you have electric heat or your heat is started electrically (an oil burner is started electrically). The heating protection is for November 15 to March 15. For more information about the documentation you would have to provide, call your utility.

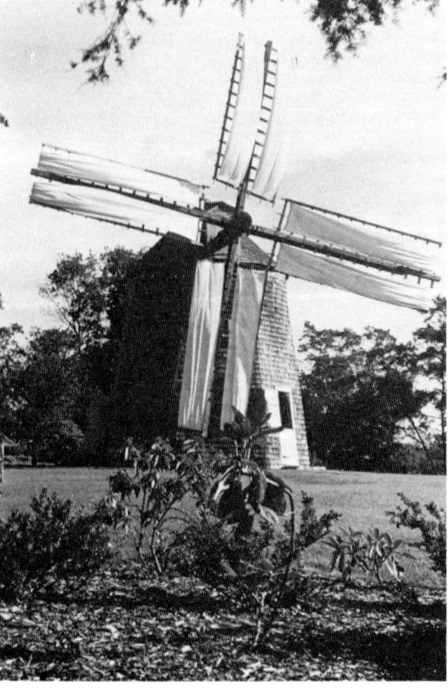

Cape Cod windmill
Eastham

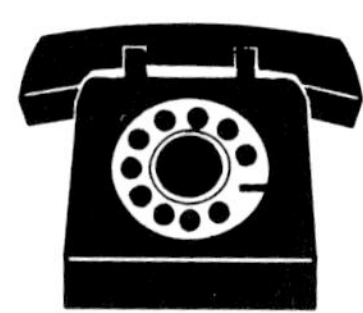

Help When You Need It

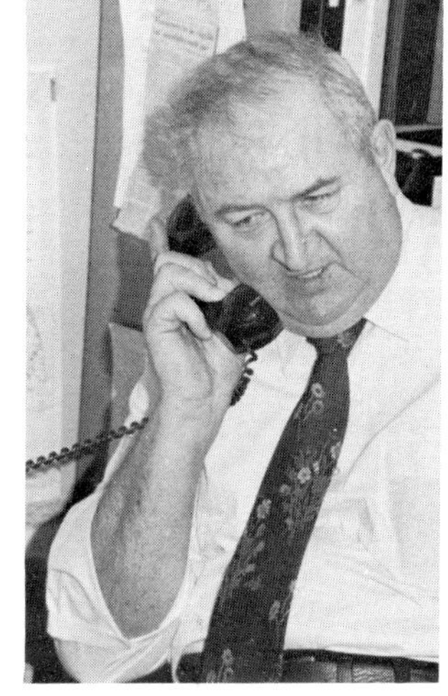

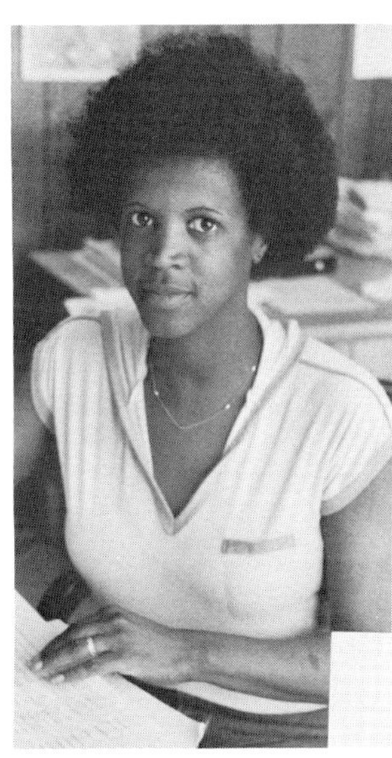

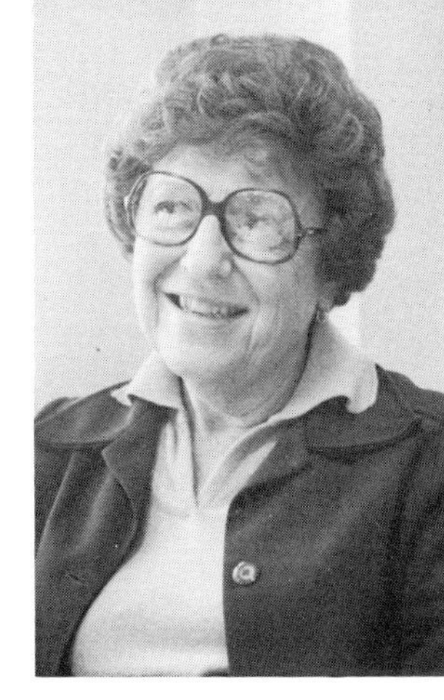

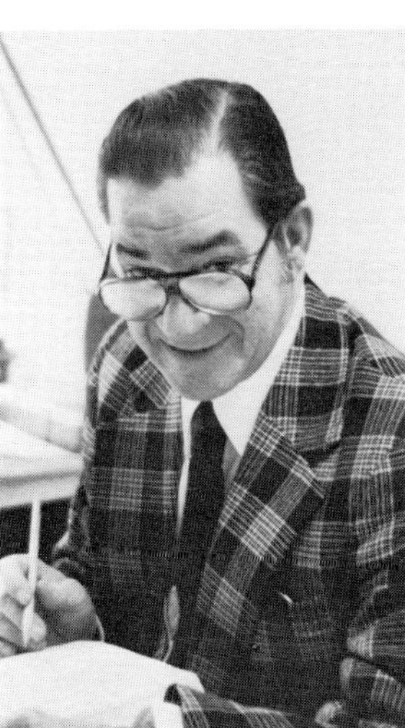

I get by with a little help from my friends.
—John Lennon & Paul McCartney

When you need more help than a friend or family can provide, there are many people to turn to in Massachusetts. Toll free numbers for legal and medical referrals, home care services, and the Elder Hot Line—Toll free **1-800-882-2003**, or **727-8931** in the Boston area—are just a few of the services available to you when you face problems that are best solved with professional help. And if your income is low, you'll find that you can still get the help you need without paying a high (or sometimes *any*) price.

Three places to call. When you need to find help in your own area, you can call the following:

- your council on aging (pp. 81-83)
- your Home Care Corporation (pp. 54-55)
- area information and referral service (p. 89)

Directories. If you are interested in a directory of service organizations in your own area, see p. 89.

An especially useful directory for the greater Boston area is the *Human Services Yellow Pages* (see p. 87).

This section includes information about:

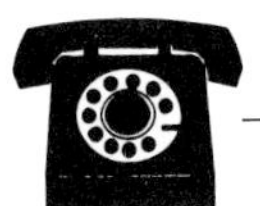

Legal advice

When you should see a lawyer

You should check with a lawyer if:

- You want to sell your home or buy a new one;
- You are signing a contract, especially with a nursing home;
- You want to make a will;
- You have tax or estate problems;
- You have to make decisions on group life insurance;
- You consider naming or changing the beneficiary of your life insurance, a private pension plan or an annuity;
- You want to give legal authority to another person.

How to find a lawyer

If you don't have a lawyer, ask friends to suggest one, or call one of the following organizations for a free referral:

Massachusetts Bar Association
Boston area: **542-9103**
Statewide: **1-800-392-6164** (toll free)
National Lawyers Guild, Mass. Chapter
(617) **227-7008**, 1–5 p.m.

Both organizations can recommend lawyers who use a sliding fee schedule and charge clients in relation to their ability to pay. The Guild specializes in helping low and moderate income people and does a limited number of cases for *very* low fees.

If you cannot afford a lawyer

There are legal offices set up all over the state that provide free legal advice to people who cannot afford to pay.

If you live *outside* the greater Boston area, call the free lawyer referral service: **1-800-392-6164** to get the location and phone number of a free legal services office near you. Some of these offices have specialists in problems of people over 60.

If you live in the Boston area, there is a special office for people 60 and over. Call to find out if they can help you:

Greater Boston Elderly Legal Services
102 Norway Street
Boston, MA 02115
536-0400

Greater Boston Elderly Legal Services will handle problems with Social Security, Supplemental Security Income, welfare, Medicaid/Medicare, utility shut-offs, landlord/tenant or consumer problems, veterans benefits, complaints about nursing homes, and other legal issues.

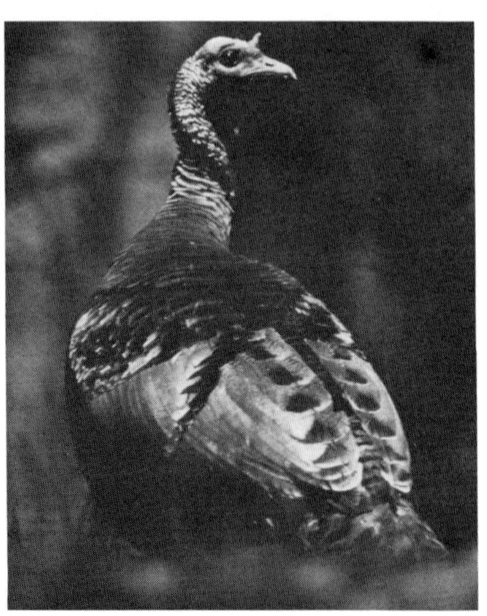

◂ **Wild turkeys** were near extinction in Massachusetts by the middle of the 19th century, but the pilgrim bird is making a comeback.

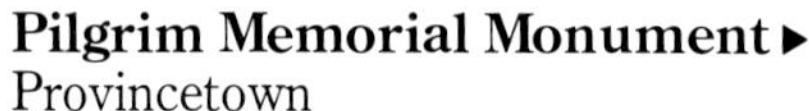

Pilgrim Memorial Monument ▸
Provincetown

Monument commemorating the landing of the Pilgrims on the outermost tip of Cape Cod, on November 11, 1620, before they reached Plymouth Rock.

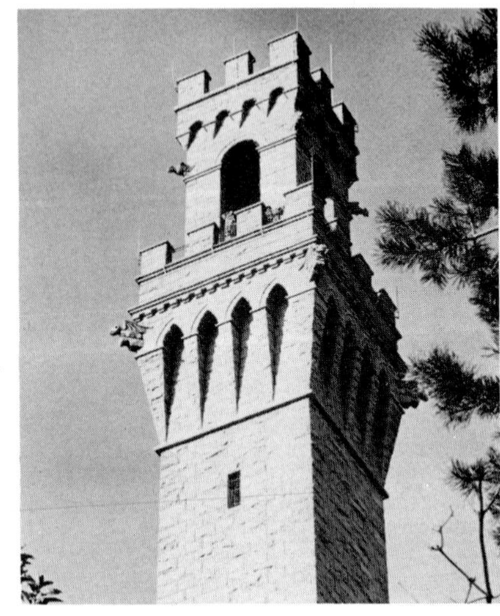

How to find a doctor or dentist

Free doctor referral

If you want the names of doctors in your area who are in general practice or who specialize (surgery, internal medicine, etc.), the Massachusetts Medical Society can help. They sponsor a free phone number for Massachusetts residents to call: **1-800-322-2303**. Boston area residents should call **536-8812**.

Free dentist referral

The Massachusetts Dental Society, in Wellesley, can give you a number to call in your own area if you want a referral to a general dentist or a dental specialist near you. There is no charge for this referral service.

(617) **237-6511** if you live near Wellesley
1-800-342-8747 (toll free) if you live elsewhere

Home care corporations

Many older people want to continue to live at home but need a bit of help with such things as cleaning, shopping or minor home repairs. Throughout Massachusetts there are non-profit Home Care Corporations which help provide that kind of assistance to people who are 60 or older and whose incomes are limited. There is a Home Care Corporation for your own area (see pp. 54-55). If you are unsure which corporation serves your city or town, call your council on aging (see pp. 81-83) or the Elder Hot Line:

1-800-882-2003 (toll free) if you live outside Boston
727-8931 if you live in the Boston area

The Home Care Corporation will help you figure out what kinds of home care you need and then make sure you get that assistance. (The care, such as a homemaker coming into your house, is actually provided by some local organization which is paid by the Home Care Corporation). These are examples of the kind of help you could get:

Chore services—snow removal, minor home repairs, heavy household cleaning, preparing for a move.

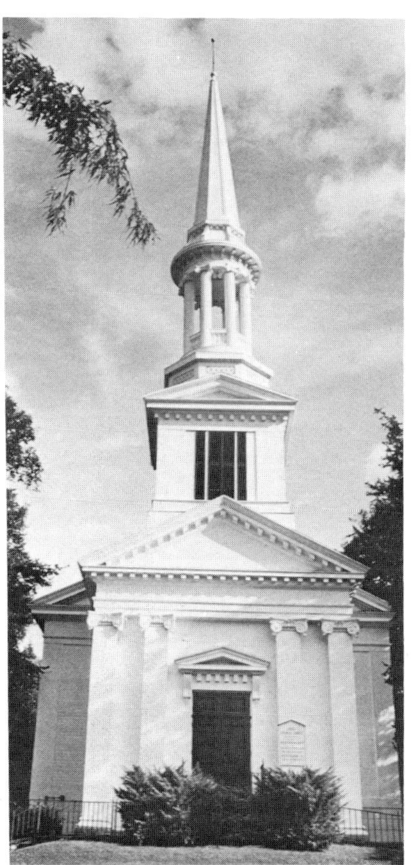

◂ **First Church of Christ**
Sandwich

This beautiful church houses an antique organ and a church bell believed to be the oldest in America.

Plimoth Plantation ▸
Plymouth (617) 746-1622

A cooper demonstrates the way barrels were made 350 years ago in the recreated pilgrim colony. See No. 11, p.65.

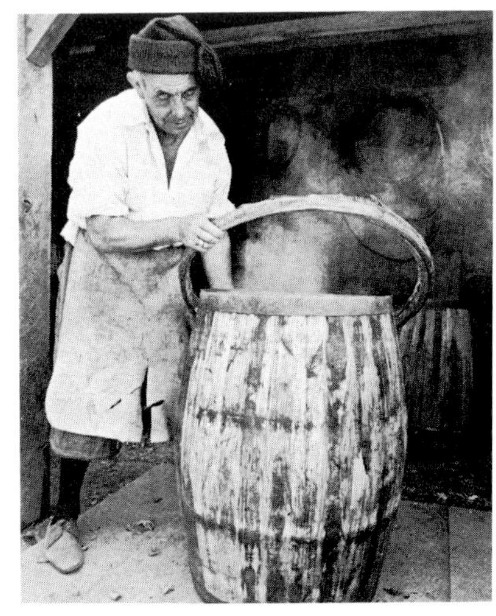

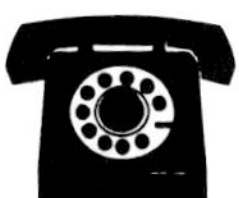

Homemaker services—including food shopping, personal errands, cooking meals, and light housekeeping.
Transportation services—help in getting to medical appointments, community service agencies, or other places.
Emergency services—counseling and other help in times of crisis.
Information and Referrals—information about where to get help—this assistance is available to all older people *regardless of income.*

Other services currently available* include: companionship, laundry, home delivered meals ("meals on wheels"), respite care, and social day care.

To be eligible for service free of charge, you must be 60 or over and have a basic annual income of not more than $7,604 for 1 person, or $10,676 for 2 people.

Other people with slightly higher incomes can receive home care services for a small fee. For a single person with an annual income between $7,605-9,067, the monthly charge varies from $8-16 according to the services provided. For a couple with an income between $10,677-11,846, the charge is between $14-23.

Services will *not* be stopped if you are unable to pay the fee.

*As of August 1985

Directory of Home Care Corporations

(Call the office nearest you)

Boston, Cambridge, Somerville

Southwest Boston Senior Services
Hyde Park, South Jamaica Plain, Roslindale, West Roxbury, Mattapan
325-6565

Central Boston Elder Services
(Allston, Back Bay, Brighton, Fenway, Jamaica Plain, North Dorchester, Parker Hill, Roxbury, South End)
Boston
266-1672

Senior Home Care Services, Boston III
(Beacon Hill, West End, Charlestown, China-town, Columbia Point, Dorchester, East Boston, East Mattapan, North End, South Boston)
Boston
451-6400

Somerville/Cambridge Elder Services
Somerville
628-2601

West of Boston

Minuteman Home Care Corporation
Lexington
862-6200

West Suburban Elder Services
West Newton
969-0170

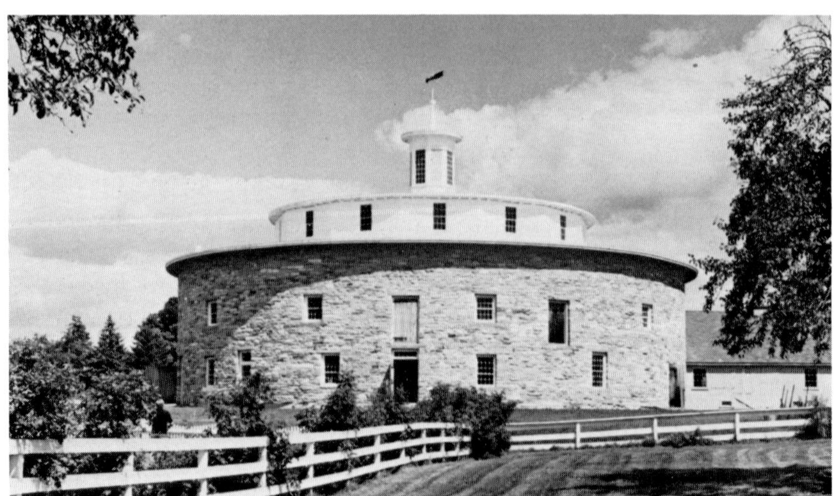

Shaker Village
Hancock (413) 443-0188

The Round Stone Barn was built in 1826 and is an example of Shaker practicality. See No. 75, p.69.

Baypath Senior Citizens Services
Framingham
620-0840

North of Boston

Senior Home Care Services
Gloucester
281-1750

North Shore Elder Services
Peabody
535-6220

Greater Lynn Senior Services
Lynn
599-0110

Elder Services of the Merrimack Valley
Lawrence
683-7747; 1-800-892-0890 (toll free)

Chelsea/Revere/Winthrop
Home Care Center
Revere
286-0550

Mystic Valley Elder Services
Malden
324-7705

South of Boston

King Phillip Elder Services
Foxborough
543-2611

South Shore Home Care Services
Braintree
848-3910

Old Colony Elderly Services
Brockton
584-1561

Southeast, Cape Cod

Bristol County Home Care for Elderly
Fall River
675-2101

Coastline Elderly Services
New Bedford
998-3016

Elder Services of Cape Cod and the Islands
West Yarmouth
771-4248

Central Massachusetts

Region II Area Agency on Aging
Holden
829-5364

Montachusett Home Care Corporation
Fitchburg
345-7312

Elder Home Care Services of Worcester Area
Worcester
756-1545

Tri-Valley Elder Services
Southbridge
764-2501

Western Massachusetts

Elder Services of Berkshire County
Pittsfield
499-1353

Franklin County Home Care Corporation
Turners Falls
774-2994

Highland Valley Elder Service Center
Northampton
586-2000; 1-800-322-0551

Holyoke/Chicopee Regional Senior Services
Holyoke
538-9020

Home Care Corporation of Springfield
Springfield
781-8800

Other home care providers

If your income is too high for you to get home care through a Home Care Corporation, the Corporation can still refer you to other sources of assistance. Available services and charges will vary from area to area. Another good source of information is your council on aging (see pp. 81-83).

Visiting Nurse Associations and other certified home health agencies provide nursing care at home for those who need it. They are independent organizations and may serve one or more communities. For example, the Visiting Nurse Association of Boston also services Chelsea, Revere and Winthrop. Your doctor or hospital can refer you to the Visiting Nurse Association or home health agency that serves people in your area.

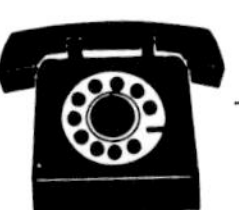

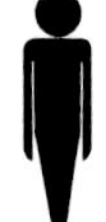

Taking care of yourself

Eating well

Nutrition Information is available free from the Massachusetts Nutrition Resource Center in Boston. A registered dietician will answer nutrition questions over the phone, send you helpful pamphlets, and make referrals to nutrition resources. You may obtain a free senior nutrition information packet, as well as choose from among 50 other free fact sheets on nutrition, such as high fiber, low salt, and low fat diets. Call the Nutrition Hotline **1-800-322-7203** (toll free) from 9 a.m. to 3 p.m. Monday through Friday. Or write:

Massachusetts Nutrition Resource Center
150 Tremont Street
Boston, MA 02111

Help yourself to a hot meal for little or nothing

The federal government presently funds nutrition projects to provide hot meals for people 60 years and over. In some areas, people who are unable to go out can have a meal delivered hot to their home.

The nutrition sites (places where the meals are served) are generally located in schools, churches, or community centers. At present there are 27 nutrition projects which serve meals daily at over 280 sites throughout the state.

The amount you pay for a meal varies from nothing to $1.00. This depends on the town or area you live in and the amount of funding your local project has received.

If you live *in Boston* and want to find out about a nutrition site near you, call the Elderly Hotline: **722-4646.** If you live *outside* the Boston area, call your local council on aging (see pp. 81-83) or your city or town Board of Health.

Smoking/Nonsmoking

If you smoke. Even if you have smoked for many years, **stopping** is the right thing for your health. For tips and support in quitting, and for referrals to other sources of help, you can call your local hospital or the hotline (formerly the "Smoker's Quitline") maintained by the Cancer Information Service: **1-800-422-6237** (toll free).

If you do not smoke, you may nevertheless be inhaling **second-hand smoke**, which recent research has shown to be harmful to non-smokers. **Protect yourself**. Ask others around you not to smoke, try to get organizations you belong to and your employer to discourage smoking, ask to sit in a non-smoking area in a restaurant.

For everyone. Avoiding inhaling smoke is particularly important if you have a heart or lung ailment.

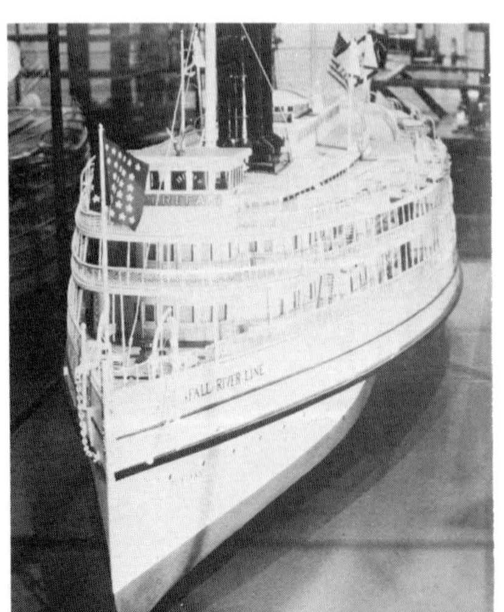

◂ **Marine Museum**
Fall River (617) 674-3533

One of the many intricate scale models housed in the museum. See No. 9, p.65.

Connecticut Valley Historical Museum ▸
Springfield (413) 732-3080

History of valley residents from 1630 to the present. Ask about the "History to Go" program. See No. 64, p.68.

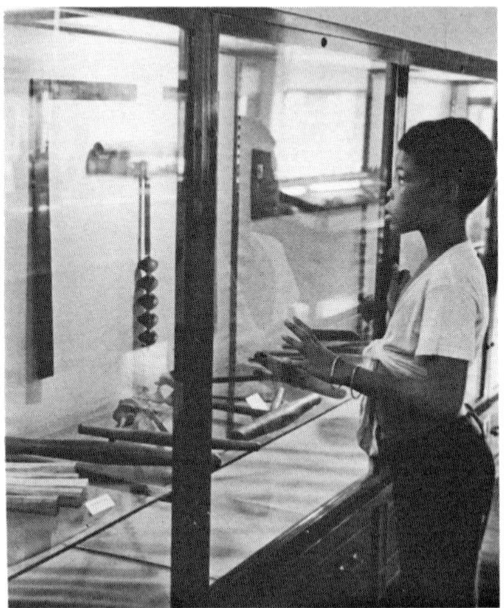

Cancer

Cancer Information Service (1-800-422-6237, toll-free) offers information about cancer and what to do about it: prevention, detection, treatment, rehabilitation, and continuing care. They can suggest treatment centers as well as services such as home health care, support groups, and even transportation that might be needed. Their free publication, "Cancer Facts For People Over 50", written especially for older people, is available by calling the toll free number above.

If your hearing is impaired

The Massachusetts Office of Deafness has information and special help for people who are hearing impaired. Call them at:

Voice (617) **727-5106**
TDD/TTY only, (617) **727-5236**
V/TDD 1-800-882-1155 (toll free)

Or write: **Mass. Office of Deafness**
20 Park Plaza
Boston, MA 02116

Blindness or sight impairments

Information, referrals, and other kinds of help are available from:

Mass. Association for the Blind
(617) **738-5510**
1-800-682-9200 (toll free)

Vision Foundation
(617) **926-4232**
1-800-852-3029 (toll free)

Mass. Commission for the Blind
(State agency for people who are legally blind)
(617) **727-5500**
1-800-392-6450 (toll free)

Large print books

Many books now are available in large print editions. Ask your librarian if they are kept in a special section. The Boston Public Library has a special catalog of its large type books. If you are looking for a specific title, your librarian may be able to find it for you in the large type books section of "Books in Print." If your library doesn't have the book, it may be available from another library through the interlibrary loan system.

"Talking" books

There is a growing collection of books recorded on tape cassettes. Your library may have some. Tape recorded books are also sold commercially. One company with a large selection is Books on Tape; you can call them toll free for a brochure at: **1-800-626-3333.** Recorded books and playback equipment are also available from the Library of Congress, free of charge and postage free, to blind and physically handicapped people. Write to:

National Library Service for the Blind and Physically Handicapped
Library of Congress
Washington, D.C. 20542

Special telephone equipment

There are many products now on the market to make telephoning easier for people with hearing, speech, vision, or motion impairments. They range from phones with volume boosters for speaking or listening, large letter dials or buttons, or visual signals for ringing, to an electronic artificial larynx, a special coupler for someone who wears a hearing aid, and various portable communications devices. One major source of special equipment is:

AT&T National Special Needs Center
2001 Route 46
Parsippany NJ 07054
1-800-233-1222 (toll free) voice
1-800-833-3232 (toll free) TDD/TTY

Seeing or hearing dogs

Of the many helpful things available to people with sight or hearing impairments, a specially trained dog may be among the most welcome. Information about seeing eye dogs is available from organizations listed elsewhere on this page. To find out more about getting a dog specially trained to help a person who is deaf or has a serious hearing impairment, contact this non-profit organization:

Red Acre Farm Hearing Dog Center
109 Red Acre Road—Box 278
Stow, MA 01775
(617) **897-8343** (voice/TTY)
(617) **897-5370** (voice only)

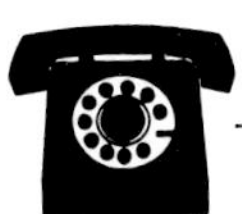

Special transportation

In an emergency

Call your Police Department. Almost all cities and towns have an emergency vehicle and team that they provide free of charge.

For the handicapped

Some cities and towns offer transportation to people who are unable to use regular public transit vehicles. Call your city or town hall for more information.

The MBTA's **"The Ride"**, for people who can't use regular transportation, is available in fourteen area cities and towns: **Arlington, Belmont, Boston, Brookline, Cambridge, Chelsea, Everett, Malden, Medford, Newton, Revere, Somerville, Watertown,** and **Winthrop**. Phone **722-5123** or **TDD/TTY 722-5415**. See p. 24 for more information.

Non-profit "multi-service" organizations

There are many private, non-profit organizations that provide several different kinds of help. Many offer assistance to people of all ages, but frequently a multi-service organization is specially interested in helping older people. Your council on aging, home care corporation (see pp. 54-55), priest, minister or rabbi probably will know about the organizations in your area.

One long-established multi-service organization for the greater Boston area is the Women's Educational and Industrial Union. The Union serves men and women of all ages. It operates shops, some of which accept handiwork on consignment; it has a career services department that maintains job listings and helps people find work; it runs support groups for older workers; and it also coordinates homemaker and home health aide placement (upon agency and private referrals). The Union runs a "Companions Unlimited" program that provides transportation to and from medical appointments, shopping and other services for shut-ins. And the Union also offers lectures and programs for everyone. Call **536-5651** or write:

Women's Educational & Industrial Union
356 Boylston Street
Boston, MA 02116

Alcohol problems

For information about help available in your area:

Alcohol Information and Referral
1-800-272-2586 (toll free)
8 a.m. to 10 p.m. weekdays
(617) **524-7884,** 24 hours a day

Mental health problems

For information about help available in your area:

Mass. Association for Mental Health
1-800-392-6135 (toll free)

United Way of Massachusetts Bay
(617) **482-1454**

If you feel lonely, despairing, or suicidal

The Samaritans are available 24 hours a day, seven days a week. Feel free to call **any** of the Samaritans' numbers:

Metropolitan Boston	(617) **247-0220**
Framingham	(617) **875-4500**
Falmouth	(617) **548-8900**
Fall River	(617) **636-6111**
Lawrence	(617) **688-6607**
Providence, R.I.	(401) **272-4044**
Keene, N.H.	(603) **357-5505**

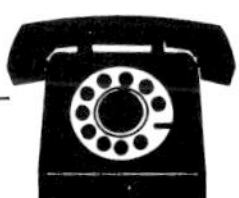

Caring for someone else

Many of the resources in this book will be helpful to you if you are helping to care for someone else. If that person is quite elderly or is suffering from Alzheimer's or a similar disease, you will be interested in an especially helpful book, *The 36-Hour Day*, by Mace and Rabins (Johns Hopkins U. Press), an unusual combination of practical information about the "mechanics" of difficult care situations and valuable insights and advice concerning your own feelings and needs as a caregiver.

Home health care supplies

You may be able to find the things you need at your pharmacy, surgical supply store, or other local retailer. Another good source may be a mail order house, from which you can order out of a catalog. Sears, for instance, has a special *Home Health Care Catalog* which you can get from:

Sears Roebuck & Company
Attention: Dept. 139
201 Brookline Avenue
Boston, MA 02215

Two other catalogs of interest are listed on p. 40. Also see the directories and information and referral services mentioned on pp. 87 and 89.

A portable telephone

One of the nicest things to give someone whose mobility is limited is a portable telephone they can have nearby wherever they may be—in bed, in a wheelchair, in a chair in another room, etc. Available in phone stores and elsewhere, this type of phone usually must be placed on its cradle for a certain number of hours a day to recharge its battery.

Special help if someone is dying

Is someone in your family terminally ill? Having "**hospice**" care could make a big difference. Hospice care is provided by a skilled team, headed by a physician, specially trained to help meet the needs of terminally ill patients **and** their families. The care can often be provided regardless of where the dying person is—at home, in a hospital, or in a nursing home or other care facility. The aim of hospice care is to improve the quality of life for terminally-ill patients and their families. A hospice team can provide a variety of services and trained personnel such as skilled nurses, home health aides, and supportive counselors for patients and their families.

There are now approximately 20 hospice teams serving 80 communities in Massachusetts. More are being formed all the time. You can find out if there is a hospice team in your area by asking your physician, your hospital, or your local Visiting Nurse Association, or by calling the Cancer Information number **1-800-422-6237** (toll free).

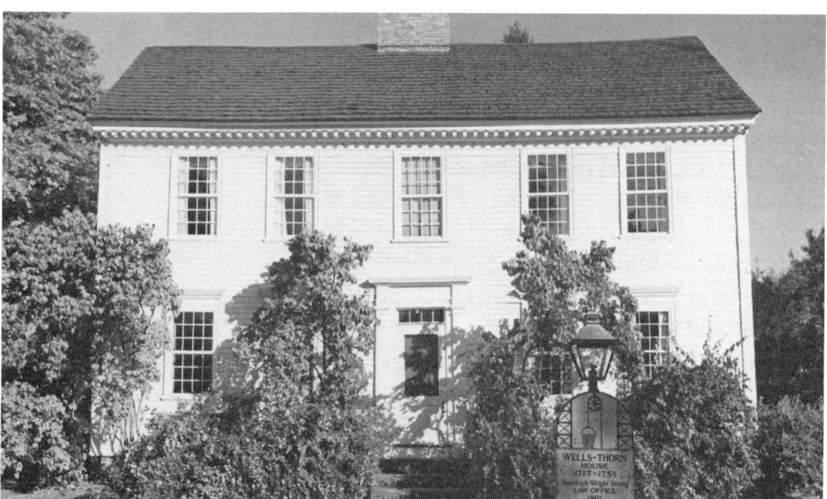

The Wells-Thorn House
Deerfield (413) 774-5581

One of ten historic houses maintained by the Historic Deerfield Foundation, the Wells-Thorn House dates from 1717. See No. 71, p.69.

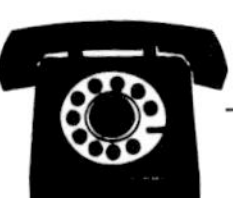

When a loved one dies

It is always a good idea to ask the advice of relatives, friends, or people at your place of worship who have had to make funeral and burial arrangements. They can help steer you to reputable people and give you an idea of costs.

To help pay for the burial, Social Security pays a lump sum of $255. Call your Social Security office with the following information at hand: your spouse's or relative's Social Security number, date of birth, and date of death.

The $255 **burial benefit** from Social Security is available if the deceased either fully qualified for Social Security checks or had been covered by Social Security for 1½ of the past 3 years of employment. Payment will be made to a surviving spouse, children, or parents eligible for survivor's benefits.

Survivor's benefits may also be available. If anyone in your immediate family was getting Social Security checks *or* had been working long enough to be eligible for checks, you should call Social Security. (See pages 5–6 for more on Social Security.)

For the funeral and burial of a veteran, $150 is available from the Veterans' Administration (see p.15). As an alternative, veterans may be buried in the Massachusetts National Cemetery at Otis Air Force Base, Cape Cod.

The Massachusetts Memorial Society of New England provides information on plans for simple funerals, and guides members to sympathetic and cooperative funeral directors. It has a 24-hour answering service: (617) **731-2073.** Or, for more information, write:

Memorial Society of New England
25 Monmouth Street
Brookline, MA 02146

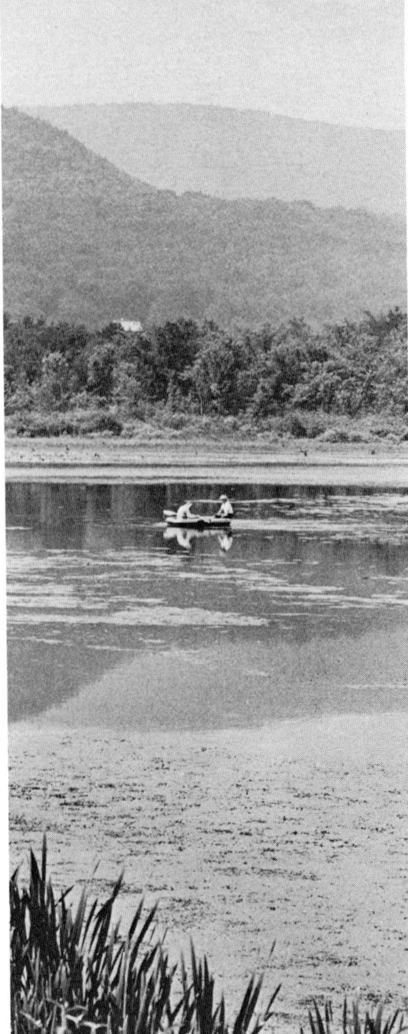

Pontoosuc Lake
Lanesboro

A year-round recreation area.

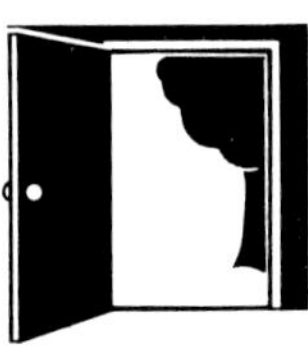

Going Places

My heart is warm with the friends
I make,
And better friends I'll not be knowing;
Yet there isn't a train I wouldn't take,
No matter where it's going.
—Edna St. Vincent Millay

There is an extraordinary number of things to do and places to go in Massachusetts. The pictures in this book give you just a sample. Many places offer free admission or special discounts. You can find out by calling in advance or asking when you go, by calling your local council on aging for places in your own community (see pp. 81-83), or by looking at the list on pp. 65-69.

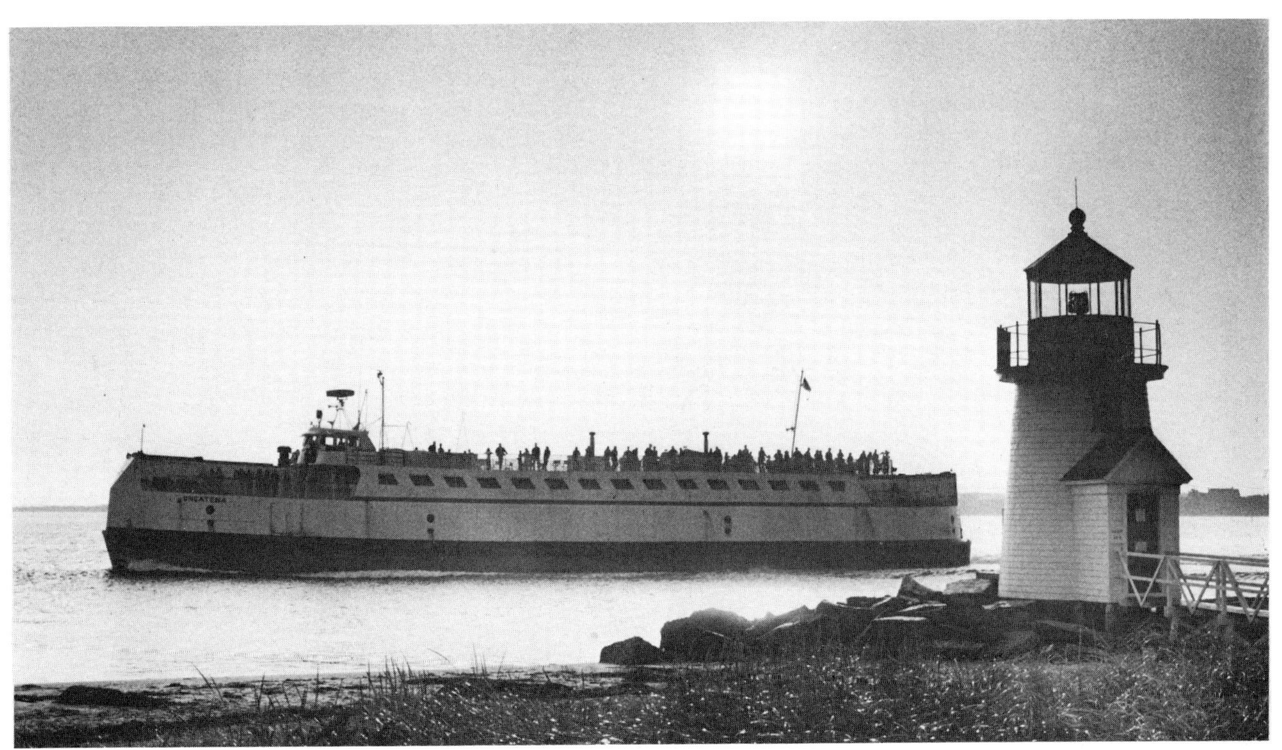

The next few pages cover:

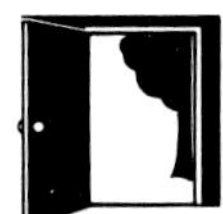

Massachusetts—a great place to visit, even if you live here

For *free publications* on things to do and places to go in Massachusetts and for a calendar of events or the official state map, write:

Division of Tourism
Department of Commerce and Development
100 Cambridge Street, 13th floor
Boston, MA 02202
(617) **727-3201**

There are also **tourist information centers** on the Mass. Pike at several of the rest areas, both eastbound and westbound.

If you are a lover of **theatre, dance, and music,** Arts/Boston issues a free booklet that lists performances in the Boston area for which you can get tickets at half price. Call (617) **423-4454** to get on the mailing list for the booklet. You can get your tickets by mail, too. Half price tickets for major shows are also available from Bostix, at their booth at Quincy Market, *on the day of the show.*

Country fairs are fun to go to, and a list of where and when they will be held is published late in the spring each year. For a listing of all the agricultural fairs in Massachusetts, send a self-addressed, long (business sized) envelope, with 28¢ postage on it, to:

Division of Fairs
Department of Food and Agriculture
100 Cambridge Street
Boston, MA 02202

Antiques. Massachusetts is a great place to look for antiques. The yellow pages of your telephone directory list antique dealers in your area. Newspapers print information about antique shows and estate sales.

State-owned recreational facilities. All state parks, beaches, and other recreational facilities are free to people over 62 with an identity card. Write for a Senior Citizen's Pass, enclosing a copy of your birth certificate or a copy of your driver's license:

Division of Forestry and Parks
Department of Environmental Management
100 Cambridge Street
Boston, Massachusetts 02202
(617) **727-3180**

In addition to 33 state parks, Massachusetts has 21 state beaches and reservations and 47 state forests. Activities and facilities range from swimming and boating to camping, fishing, nature trails and simply strolling in beautiful surroundings.

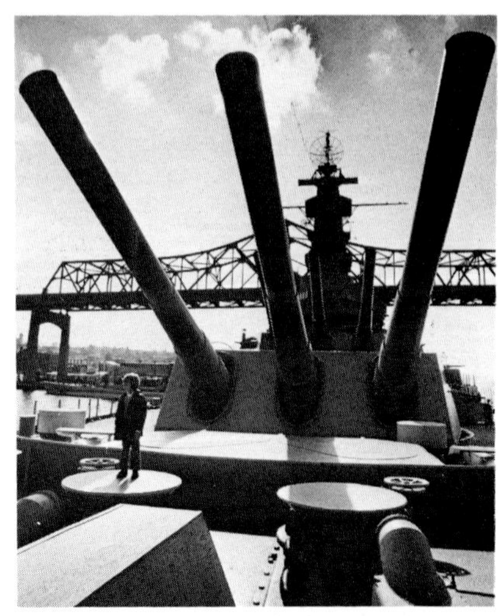

Battleship Cove
Fall River (617) 678-1100

The battleship U.S.S. Massachusetts will take you back to World War II when the ship was manned by a crew of 2,300. See No. 8, p.65.

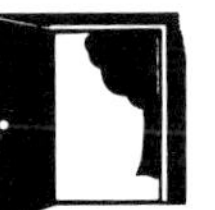

Brochures and maps are available from the state office listed above.

Metropolitan District Commission facilities. At MDC parks, skating rinks, swimming pools, and other facilities in Boston and area communities, there are special discounts, as much as 50% off for people over 65. Bring a driver's license or other proof of age with you. In the Boston area call **727-5215** for hours and information.

National Park Service facilities. The Service has a variety of parks, historic sites, and other facilities you may want to visit (Cape Cod National Seashore, or Adams National Historic Site in Quincy, for example). At parks and sites which charge admission, if you drive in, there is no entrance fee for yourself or anyone in your car, if you are 62 or over. If you walk in, there is no entrance fee for yourself or anyone with you who is in your immediate family if you are at least 62. Within the Park Service area, camping and other park fees are half price for people 62 or over.

Go to the park with a birth certificate or driver's license and ask for a Golden Age Pass, or you can get the pass in advance at the Park Service office (see below). The pass is free and never expires. It is also accepted at U.S. Fish and Wildlife locations, U.S. Foreign Service areas and U.S. Corps of Engineers sites.

The Park Service will send you a free listing of their parks and historic sites and a folder on the Golden Age Pass if you contact them at:

National Park Service
15 State Street
Boston, MA 02109
(617) **223-0058**

Two nonprofit organizations maintain open spaces and wildlife sanctuaries across Massachusetts that are open to the public. There is a nominal fee at some sites. Call or write them for a brochure listing these special places:

Massachusetts Audubon Society
South Great Road
Lincoln, MA 01773
(617) **259-9500**

Trustees of Reservations
224 Adams Street
Milton, MA 02186
(617) **698-2066**

Senior centers and churches or temples often arrange special trips and outings to interesting places. These excursions usually cost very little. Many senior centers and churches or temples also have clubs or special programs for older people. They offer all kinds of fun—movies, card games, bingo, crafts, etc. and are a great place to meet new friends. Call your city or town hall or local council on aging (see pp. 81-83) to find out about the Senior Centers, and call your place of worship and ask about activities that you might enjoy.

Libraries are another source of activity. In addition to lending books and having more magazines than you could possibly read, libraries often show movies, let you listen to music or recorded plays, and have special programs on many different topics. You might even suggest your own topic for a program. A list of suggested magazines and books is on pages 86-87.

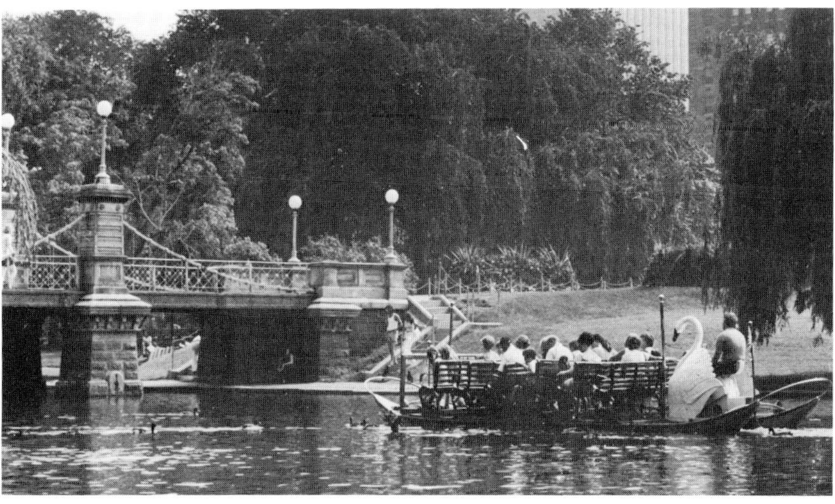

Swan Boats
Boston Public Garden

A favorite Boston experience.

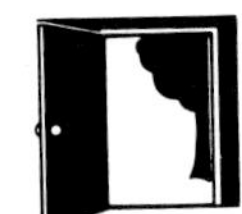

Bus tours. One of the best ways to see things in Massachusetts is by bus. A big bus can hold about 50 people, and you can take a pre-arranged tour or organize one of your own. Call a tour bus line in your area, a travel agent, or a tour broker. Among the tour brokers in various parts of Massachusetts are the following members of the National Tour Brokers Association:

Arnold Tours, Cambridge
Beckham Travel, Canton
Butler Travel Tours, N. Chelmsford
Cape Tours, Dennisport
Crimson Travel, Cambridge
Collette Travel, c/o Young's Travel, Worcester
Downtown Travel, Boston
Paragon Travel, New Bedford
Peter Pan Tours, Springfield
Valadio, Taunton

Fall foliage trains. The Mystic Valley Railway Society organizes tours by train through the peak of autumn foliage, usually Columbus Day weekend. Destinations and prices vary. For information contact:

Mystic Valley Railway Society
Box 486
Hyde Park, MA 02136
(617) **361-4445**

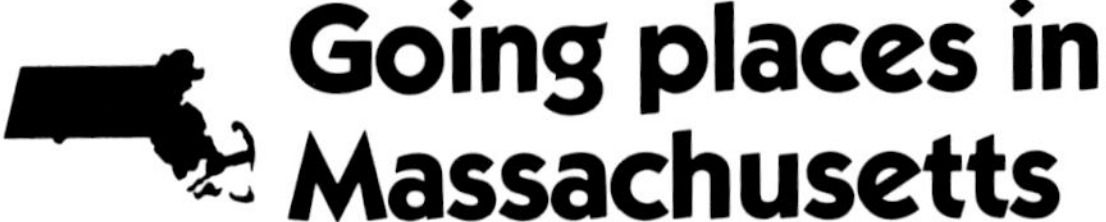

Going places in Massachusetts

If you had the time, you could make touring Massachusetts a full-time, year-round activity. The information chart below will help you decide where and when to begin your travels. The chart shows discounts for people over 65, group discounts, the season during which the attraction is open, and whether or not it is accessible to someone in a wheelchair. "Accessible" means that staff have indicated that there are ramps, no steps, or a few steps and help available.

S-F—means that the attraction is open from spring through fall. Call for exact dates.

YR —means that the attraction is open year-round.

call—means that access for handicapped people is limited or that arrangements can be made.

* —an asterisk after the listing means that there is a photograph of the place elsewhere in the book.

But call first. Almost all attractions listed here have telephones. To avoid possible disappointment because some information may have changed, you may want to call first to check dates and times when attractions are open, as well as current discount policies and accessibility.

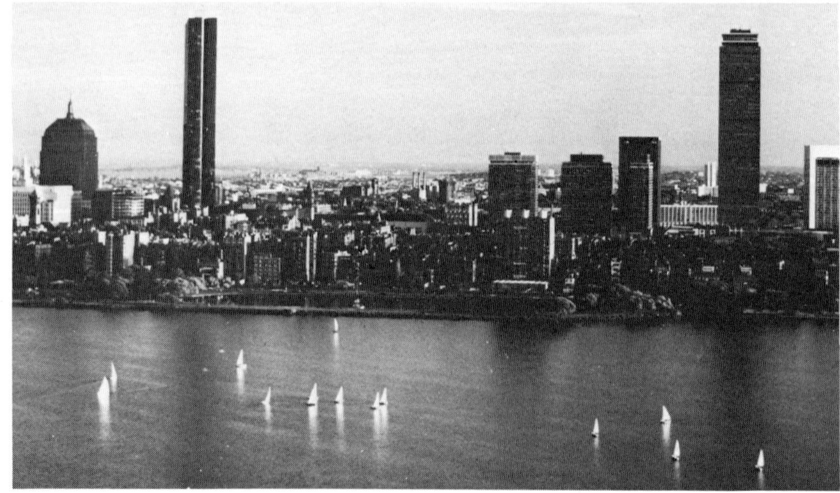

Boston skyline from the Charles River.

John Hancock Observatory
Boston (617) 247-1976
There's a great view of Boston from New England's tallest building. The Observatory includes multi-media exhibits about Boston since Revolutionary days. See No. 24, p.66.

Prudential Skywalk
Boston (617) 236-3318
See the view from the Skywalk—a garden in the sky, 50 stories above Boston. See No. 31, p.66.

	Senior Citizen Discount	Group Discount	Season	Access
Cape/Islands				
1. **The Whaling Museum** Nantucket (617) 228-1736		✓	S-F	✓
2. **The Lobster Hatchery** Martha's Vineyard (617) 693-0060	free	free	June–Aug	✓
3. **Dexter's Grist Mill** Sandwich, no telephone			S-F	✓
4. **Heritage Plantation*** Sandwich (617) 888-3300		✓	S-F	✓
5. **Sandwich Glass Museum*** Sandwich (617) 888-0251		✓	YR except Mar.	✓
Southeast				
6. **Fort Phoenix** historic site Fairhaven, no telephone	free	free	YR	✓
7. **The Whaling Museum*** New Bedford (617) 997-0046		✓	YR	call
8. **Battleship Cove*** Fall River (617) 678-1100	✓	✓	YR	
9. **Marine Museum*** Fall River (617) 674-3533	✓	✓	YR	✓
10. **Edaville Railroad*** South Carver (617) 866-4526	✓	✓	S-F	✓
11. **Plimoth Plantation*** Plymouth (617) 746-1622		✓	S-F	call
12. **Mayflower II*** Plymouth (617) 746-1622		✓	S-F	
13. **Pilgrim Hall** Plymouth (617) 746-1620	✓	✓	YR	✓
14. **The Antiquarian House*** Plymouth (617) 746-9697		✓	S-F	call
15. **Richard Sparrow House** Plymouth (617) 747-1240	donation	donation	S-F	
16. **The Jenney Grist Mill*** Plymouth (617) 747-0811	free	free	YR	✓
17. **Capron Park Zoo*** Attleboro (617) 222-3047	free	free	YR	

	Senior Citizen Discount	Group Discount	Season	Access
Boston Area				
18. **Arnold Arboretum** Boston (617) 524-1717	free	free	YR	✓
19. **Christian Science Center*** Boston (617) 262-2300	free	free	YR	✓
20. **The Boston Tea Party Museum** Boston (617) 338-1773	✓	✓	YR	
21. **Museum Wharf**, including: **The Children's Museum** Boston (617) 426-8855	✓	✓	YR	✓
The Computer Museum Boston (617) 426-2800	✓	✓	YR	✓
22. **Franklin Park Zoo** Boston (617) 442-0991	free	free	YR	✓
23. **Isabella Stewart Gardner Museum*** Boston (617) 734-1359	donation	donation	YR	call
24. **John Hancock Observatory*** Boston (617) 247-1976	✓	✓	YR	✓
25. **Massachusetts State House*** Boston (617) 727-3676	free	free	YR	
26. **Museum of Fine Arts*** Boston (617) 267-9377	✓		YR	✓
27. **Museum of Science & Hayden Planetarium*** Boston (617) 742-6088	✓	✓	YR	✓
28. **Museum of Transportation*** Brookline (617) 522-6140	✓	✓	S–F	✓
29. **New England Aquarium*** Boston (617) 742-8870	✓	✓	YR	✓
30. **Old North Church*** Boston (617) 523-6676	free	free	YR	✓
31. **Prudential Skywalk*** Boston (617) 236-3318	✓	✓	YR	✓
32. **The Paul Revere House** Boston (617) 523-1676	✓	✓	YR	✓
33. **Trinity Church** Boston (617) 536-0944	free	free	YR	call

	Senior Citizen Discount	Group Discount	Season	Access
34. **Longfellow National Historic Site*** Cambridge (617) 876-4491	free	free	YR	call
35. **Peabody Museum** Cambridge (617) 495-2248	✓	✓	YR	✓
36. **Bunker Hill Monument** Charlestown (617) 242-5641	free	free	YR	✓
37. **U.S.S. Constitution*** Charlestown (617) 242-0543	✓	✓	YR	✓ museum
38. **J.F.K. Library Museum*** Dorchester (617) 929-4523			YR	✓
39. **Captain Robert Bennet Forbes House** Milton (617) 696-1815	Opening in 1986—please call first			
40. **Adams National Historic Site*** Quincy (617) 773-1177	✓		S-F	
41. **John Adams Birthplace*** Quincy (617) 773-1177	free	free	S-F	✓
42. **Gore Place** Waltham (617) 894-2798	✓	✓	S-F	
43. **The Giant Globe*** Wellesley (617) 235-1200	free	free	YR	✓
44. **Cardinal Spellman Philatelic Museum** Weston (617) 894-6735	free	free	YR	✓
45. **The Museum of Our National Heritage*** Lexington (617) 861-6559	free	free	YR	✓
46. **DeCordova & Dana Museum & Park** Lincoln (617) 259-8355	✓	✓	YR	
47. **Drumlin Farm Wildlife Sanctuary*** Lincoln (617) 259-9807	✓	✓	YR	
48. **Minute Man National Historical Park*** Concord (617) 484-6192	free		YR	call
49. **Garden in the Woods** Framingham (617) 877-6574	✓		S-F	

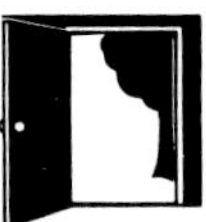

	Senior Citizen Discount	Group Discount	Season	Access
Northeast				
50. Saugus Ironworks* Saugus (617) 233-0050	free	free	S-F	✓
51. Essex Institute Historical Museum Salem (617) 744-3390	✓	✓	YR	✓
52. Lowell National Park Lowell (617) 459-1000	free	free	YR	✓
53. Salem Maritime Site Salem (617) 744-4323	free	free	YR	
54. Peabody Museum* Salem (617) 745-1876	✓		YR	✓
55. Salem Witch Museum* Salem (617) 744-1692	✓		YR	call
56. Hammond Castle* Gloucester (617) 283-2080	✓	✓	YR	
Central				
57. Fruitlands Museum Harvard (617) 456-3924		✓	summer plus	
58. John Woodman Higgins Armory* Worcester (617) 853-6015	✓	✓	YR	
59. Worcester Art Museum* Worcester (617) 799-4406	free	free	YR	✓
60. Old Sturbridge Village* Sturbridge (617) 347-3362		✓	YR	✓
Western				
61. McLaughlin State Trout Hatchery Belchertown (413) 323-7671	free	free	YR	✓
62. Laughing Brook Hampden (413) 566-8034	✓		YR	✓
63. Basketball Hall of Fame* Springfield (413) 781-6500	✓	✓	YR	✓
64. Connecticut Valley Historical Museum* Springfield (413) 732-3080	donation	donation	YR	
65. The Science Museum Springfield (413) 733-1194	donation	donation	YR	✓

	Senior Citizen Discount	Group Discount	Season	Access
66. **George Walter Vincent Smith Art Museum** Springfield (413) 733-4214	donation	donation	YR	
67. **Springfield Armory Museum*** Springfield (413) 734-8551	free	free	YR	✓
68. **Springfield Museum of Fine Arts** Springfield (413) 732-6092	donation	donation	YR	
69. **The Farm Museum** Hadley—no telephone	free	free	S-F	
70. **Leverett Craftsmen & Artists' Center** Leverett (413) 549-6871	free	free	YR	✓
71. **The Wells-Thorn House*** Deerfield (413) 774-5581		✓	YR	
72. **Chesterwood*** Stockbridge (413) 298-3579		✓	S-F	✓
73. **Norman Rockwell Museum*** Stockbridge (413) 298-3822			YR	
74. **Tanglewood*** Lenox (413) 637-1940			summer	✓
75. **Shaker Community*** Hancock (413) 443-0188	✓	✓	summer	
76. **Sterling and Francine Clark Art Institute*** Williamstown (413) 458-8109	free	free	YR	✓

Other places to visit in Massachusetts

State parks and forests. See p. 62 for more information.

National Historic Sites. Call (617) 223-0058 for information.

Audubon sanctuaries. See p. 63 for more information.

Properties of the Trustees of Reservations. See p. 63 for more information.

The Freedom Trail in Boston. Call (617) 536-4100 for maps and information.

Roxbury Heritage Trail/Black Heritage Trail in Boston. Call (617) 445-7400 for more information or write:

Museum of Afro American History
Dudley Station
Box 5
Roxbury, MA 02119

Enjoying Massachusetts

Outdoors

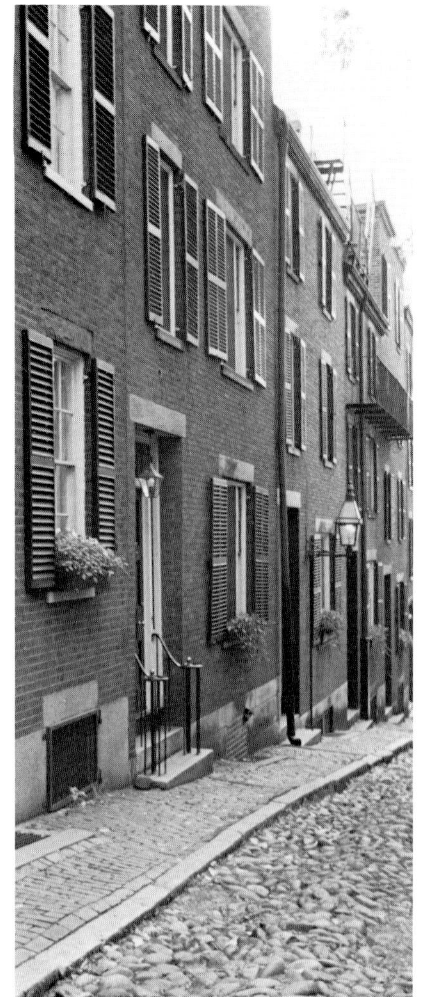

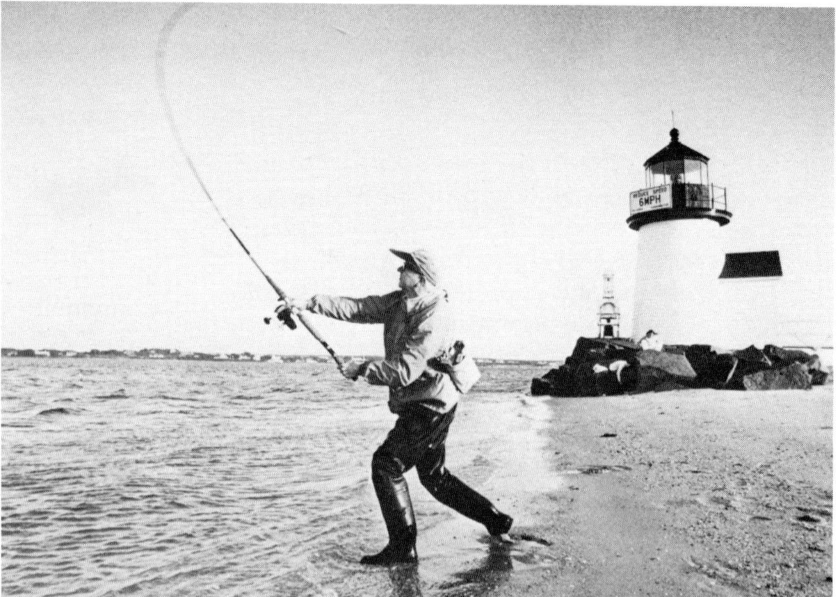

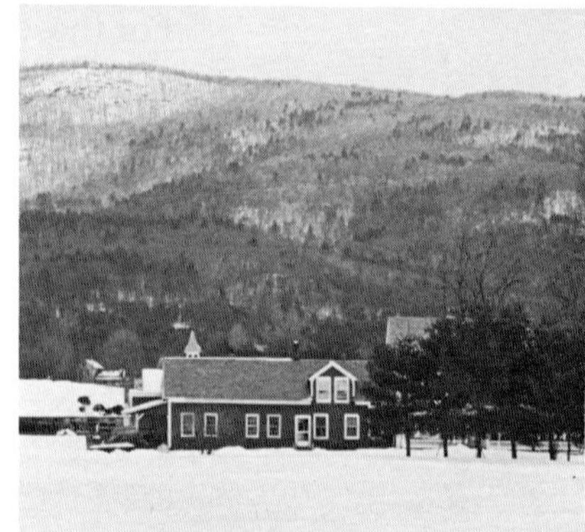

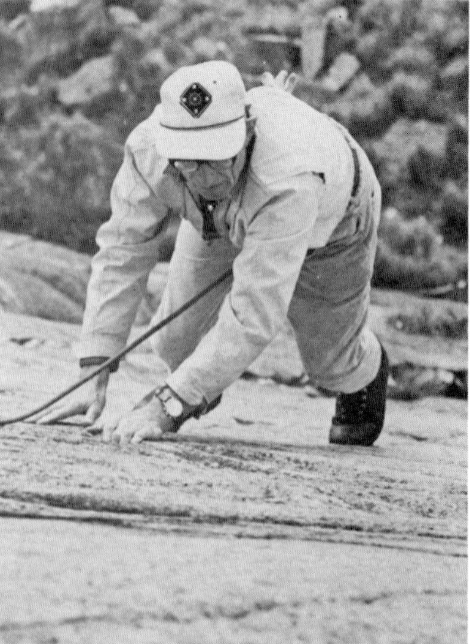

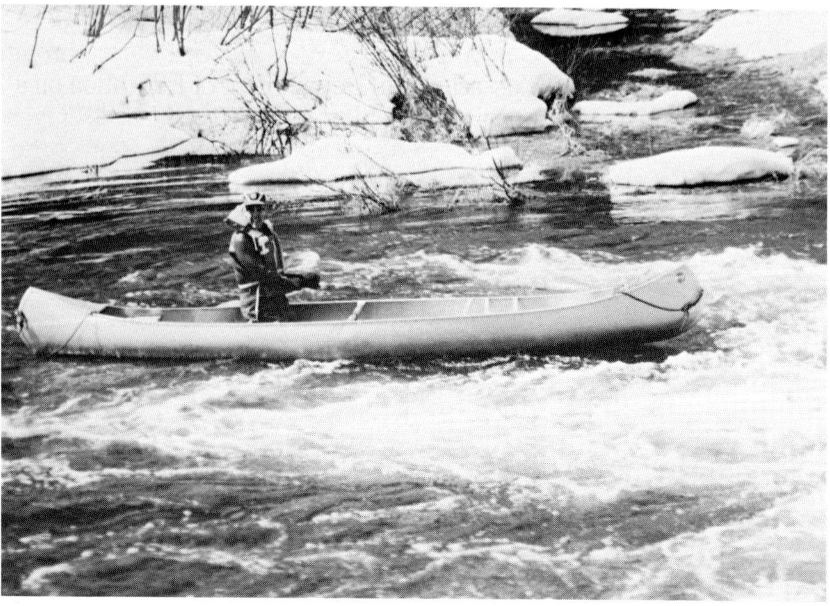

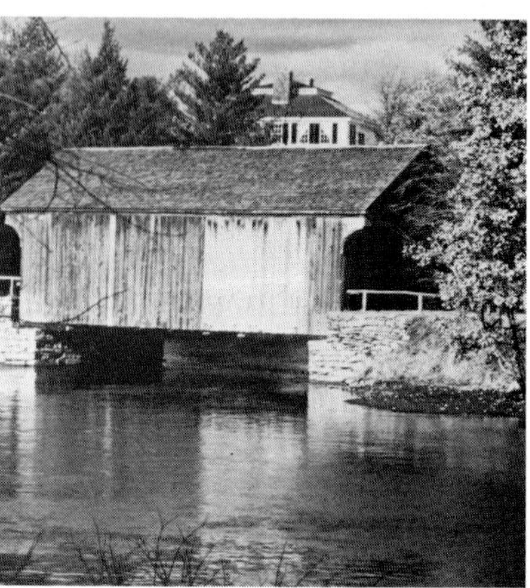

Learning something new

You can learn about art, music, history or anything that interests you *for free* in Massachusetts. State universities and community colleges charge *no* admission to residents 60 and older. Tuition paying students are given preference in a class of limited size, but space permitting, you are welcome to enroll. Call the state or community college of your choice for more information.

Almost every community has **adult education courses** that are fun and inexpensive. You can take a course on how to fix your bicycle, how to make Viennese pastries, or how to take great pictures of your grandchildren. The council on aging in your area will be able to tell you where to call about courses and fees.

If you live in the Boston area, both Middlesex Community College and the College of Public and Community Service at UMass-Boston have a Special program in gerontology (the study of aging). It will be free if you are over 60. Interested students will be able to earn a Bachelor of Arts degree or a Gerontology Certificate. Call (617) **956-1057** for more information about the gerontology program at UMass. For information about the Middlesex Community College gerontology program call (617) **275-8910**. Berkshire, Greenfield, Northern Essex and Quinsigamond Community Colleges also offer a special certificate program for older people.

If you are interested in adult basic education, GED preparation, or English-as-a-second-language programs near you, you can call:

Mass. Department of Education
Bureau of Student, Community and Adult Services
(617) **770-7580**

For those of you who live in Boston or any of its suburbs, there is a number you can call to get the names and places of courses you might want to take in your area:

The Educational Exchange of Greater Boston
1430 Massachusetts Avenue
Cambridge, MA 02138
876-3080

The Exchange also publishes a directory, *Educational Opportunities of Greater Boston*, which is likely to be available at your public library. The catalog may be purchased from the Educational Exchange for $7.95.

Correspondence courses are offered through the Massachusetts Department of Education on a great variety of subjects. If you are 65 or over, you pay only the $5 registration fee and the cost of the textbooks used in the course. For more information on the courses offered, call: (617) **770-7582** or write:

Supervisor, Correspondence Courses
Massachusetts Department of Education
1385 Hancock Street
Quincy, MA 02169

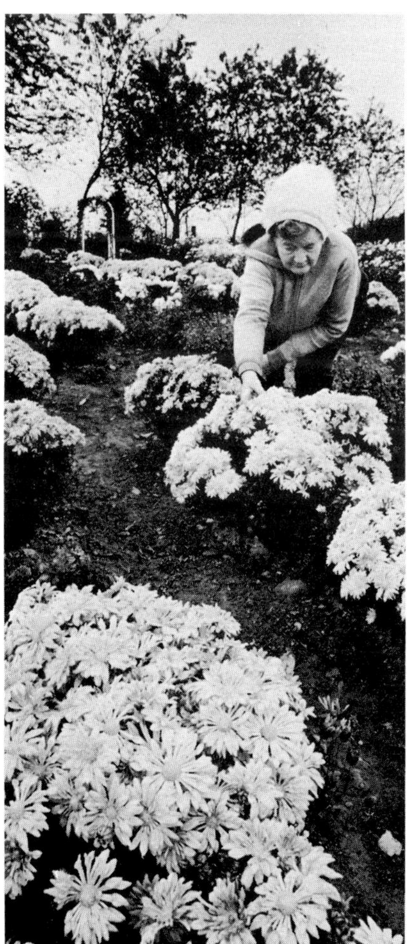

Crysanthemums
North Attleboro

Autumn is crysanthemum time in Bristol County. Dighton hosts an annual crysanthemum show.

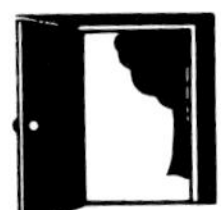

Elderhostel

Elderhostel Inc. is a network of over 700 colleges, universities and educational institutions in all 50 states and around the world, which offer academic programs for people over 60 or who attend with a spouse or a companion who is over 60. The students live in dormitories, eat in college cafeterias and attend daily classes on such subjects as the "American Civil War," "Robert Frost," "International Foods" and "The Celts and Their Culture." Sixteen Massachusetts institutions offer programs including Amherst, Emmanuel, Salem State and Williams Colleges. The courses usually last a week and in 1985 the weekly fee (including meals) is $195 per person. You don't have to have graduated from high school or college to attend. For more information, send a postcard to:

Elderhostel
80 Boylston Street, Suite 400
Boston, MA 02116

Audiovisual presentations for groups

There are many audiovisual presentations available for group showings, free or at nominal cost, on age-related subjects. For instance, the American Association of Retired Persons (AARP) makes numerous educational slide-tape programs available to organizations on a short-term loan basis at no cost except for postage to return the slides and tapes. Subjects include: consumer affairs, criminal justice services, energy, health education and advocacy, housing, and safety. All your group needs to do is get a slide projector, tape recorder, and screen. You might also want to have someone knowledgeable in the field present to add his/her comments and answer questions. For more information on obtaining presentations, contact:

AARP Area Office
823 Park Square Building
Boston, MA 02116
(617) **426-1185**

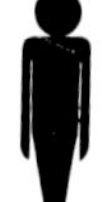

Staying in shape

If walking or jogging isn't enough exercise for you, try calling a local YMCA or YWCA about fitness programs. The Brockton YMCA and the Cambridge YWCA are just two of the Massachusetts athletic centers that offer exercise programs for older people. Your council on aging will be able to give you more suggestions (see pp. 81-83).

Museum Wharf
Boston
Home of the Children's (and grandchildren's) Museum p.66.

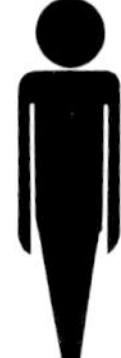

Standing Up for Your Rights

Y THE RUDE BRIDGE THAT
ARCHED THE FLOOD,
HEIR FLAG TO APRIL'S
BREEZE UNFURLED,
ERE ONCE THE EMBATTLED
FARMERS STOOD,
ND FIRED THE SHOT HEARD
ROUND THE WORLD.

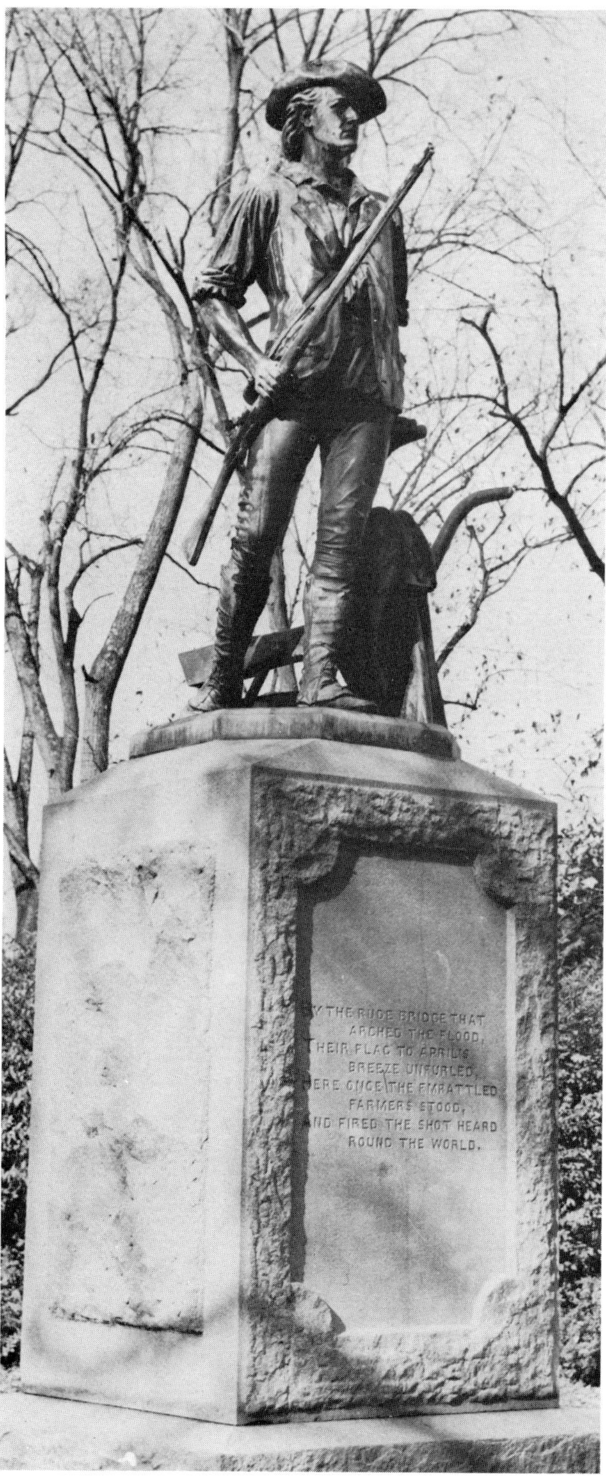

This truth keep in sight—
every man on the planet
Has just as much right as yourself
to the road.
—John Boyle O'Reilly

Many people in our society are taken advantage of or inadvertently don't get what they're entitled to—because they don't know what their legal rights are *or* just because they don't stand up for themselves. Here are brief explanations of some of your basic rights and some pointers on how to make an effective complaint.

The following pages cover:

Page

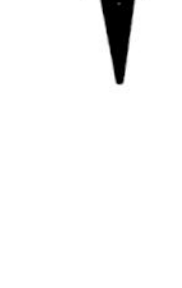

Some of your rights which are protected by Massachusetts law

Age discrimination is basically illegal. With few exceptions, Massachusetts law protects you against age discrimination in employment, credit, housing and education.

Your employment rights. If you are 40 years old or older, you are protected under Massachusetts law from discrimination because of your age, in: job advertisements, hiring, discharge, promotions, benefits or any other terms or conditions of employment. If you are at least 40 years old and believe that you have been discriminated against because of your age, you have the right to file a complaint with the Massachusetts Commission Against Discrimination (MCAD). This complaint must be filed within six months of the date that you first know of the discrimination. MCAD offices are listed on the next page.

Federal law also prohibits employment discrimination on the basis of age, but protection is limited to persons 40–69. If you wish to file a complaint pursuant to the federal law, you should contact the U.S. Equal Employment Opportunity Commission, John F. Kennedy Building, Room 409B, Boston, Massachusetts 02203. Your complaint should be filed within 180 days of the date you first know of the discrimination.

Your rights to credit. If you are over 18, no lender can refuse to grant you a mortgage loan solely on account of your age, although lenders *can* establish different terms or requirements because of an applicant's age.

A retail store that normally offers charge accounts or other forms of credit cannot refuse you those privileges only on the basis of your age.

Your housing rights. If you are over 18, you cannot be discriminated against because of your age in the sale or rental or leasing of property, and in all related real estate services such as advertising, showing of property and obtaining a mortgage.

Other important housing rights, including protection against eviction, are discussed in the housing section on p. 47.

Your rights to postgraduate and vocational education. Any postgraduate or vocational edu-

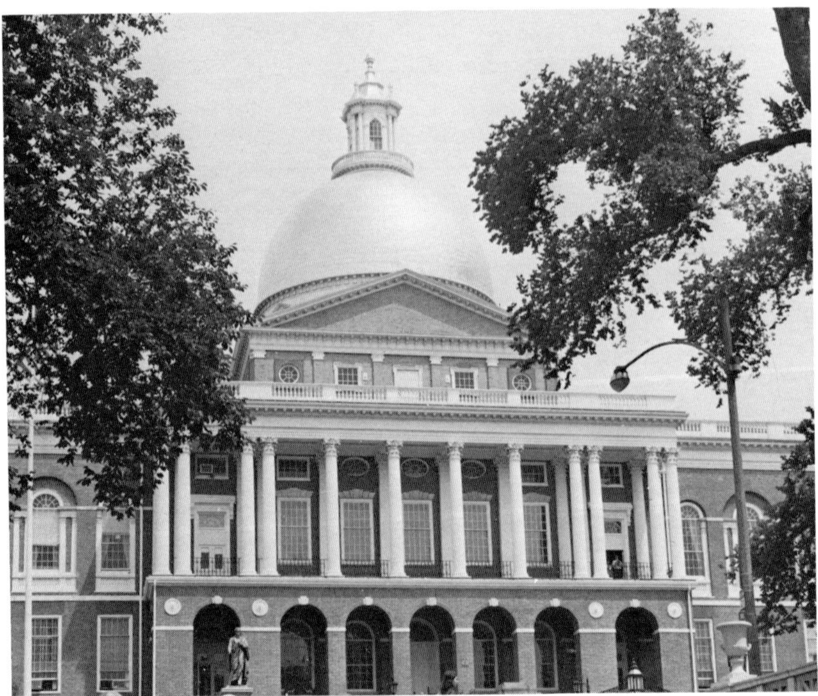

Massachusetts State House
Boston (617) 727-3676

The oldest state house still in use in the country; built in 1795 from the design of Charles Bulfinch.
See No. 25, p.66.

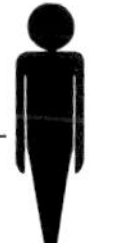

cational institution that accepts applicants from the general public may not limit, exclude or discriminate against any person because of his or her age. Students of different ages must be treated alike in any courses or programs, students' benefits or job placement programs.

If you think you might have been discriminated against

The anti-discrimination laws are more complicated than can be presented here. For more complete information about your particular situation, contact the nearest office of the Massachusetts Commission Against Discrimination (MCAD). Someone there will be glad to explain your rights more fully or help you take action against anyone who has illegally discriminated against you.

MCAD offices

Boston: Sixth Floor, One Ashburton Place (the McCormack State Office Building)
Boston, MA 02108
727-3990

Worcester: 75-A Grove Street
Worcester, MA 01605
752-2272

Springfield: 145 State Street
Springfield, MA 01103
739-3330 or **739-2145**

New Bedford 222 Union Street
New Bedford, MA 02740
997-3191

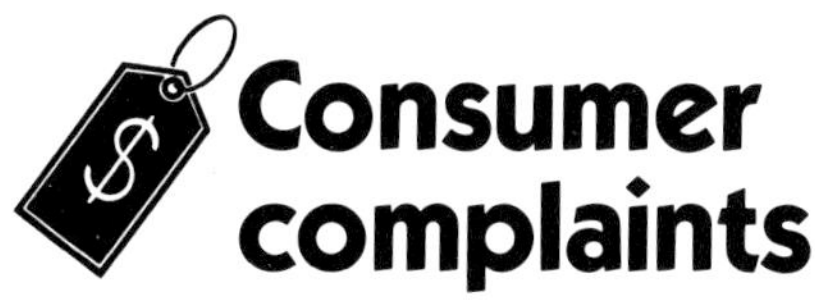

Consumer complaints

If you have a complaint about the buying or selling of goods and services, you can consult a lawyer, represent yourself in Small Claims Court, or take the complaint to your local **Consumer Council.** To find out about the Consumer Council in your area, contact your council on aging (see pp. 81-83) or write:

Department of the Attorney General
Consumer Protection Division
One Ashburton Place, Floor 19
Boston, MA 02108
(617) **727-8400**

For help with handling your complaint yourself, write:

Executive Office of Consumer Affairs
Self-Help Information Office
One Ashburton Place, Room 1411
Boston, MA 02108
(617) **727-7780**

Consumer Affairs also has publications that will interest you, including their guides to generic drugs, Medicare supplements, and funeral planning. Call the number above to get copies.

There is also a Consumer Resource Guide booklet written by the state and the Better Business Bureau that lists all kinds of consumer groups.

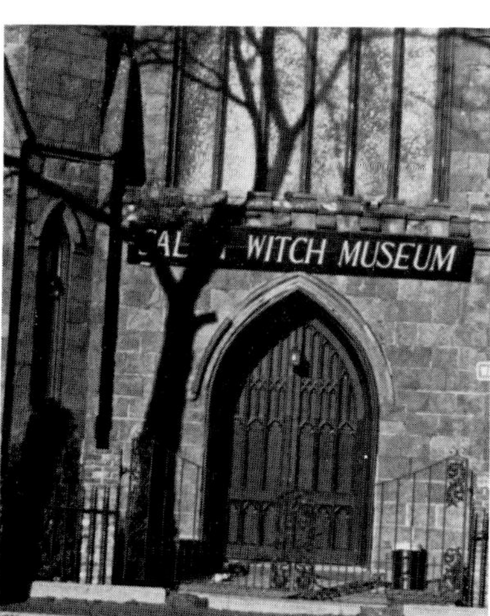

◂ **Salem Witch Museum**
Salem (617) 744-1692

Sight and sound presentation of the history of the Salem witch hunts. See No. 55, p.68.

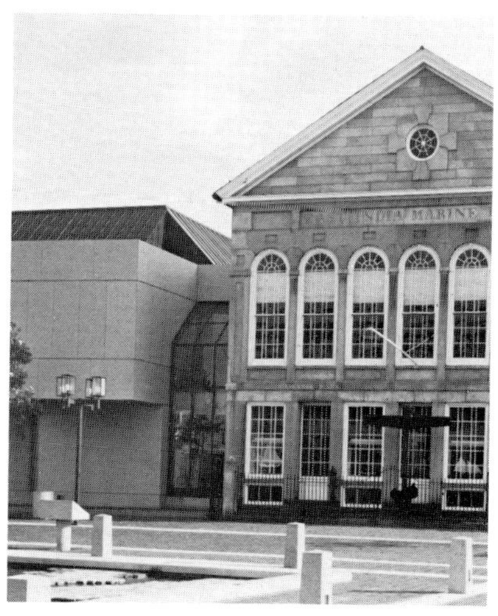

Peabody Museum ▸
Salem (617) 745-1876

Old and new buildings which exhibit "natural and artificial curiosities" brought home from around the world by sea captains. See No. 54, p.68.

You can get one by sending $3.00 (tax deductible) to:

Consumer Affairs Foundation
P.O. Box 70
Essex Station
Boston, MA 02112

Small claims court

You can sue for amounts up to $1,200 in Small Claims Court. It's not hard to do, and you will have your claim decided by a judge.

Call the courthouse nearest you and ask for the "Small Claims Department." They will tell you how to file a claim.

Tips about making a complaint

Some general advice about making a complaint—

1. Make the complaint as specific as possible: cite as many facts as you can, and know what you want to get in the end.
2. Keep a record of all the people you have spoken to and the dates you spoke to them.
3. Keep a copy of any complaint letter you send and any letters you receive.
4. When you call in response to a letter that has been sent to you, ask for the person who signed the letter you received.
5. Be persistent.

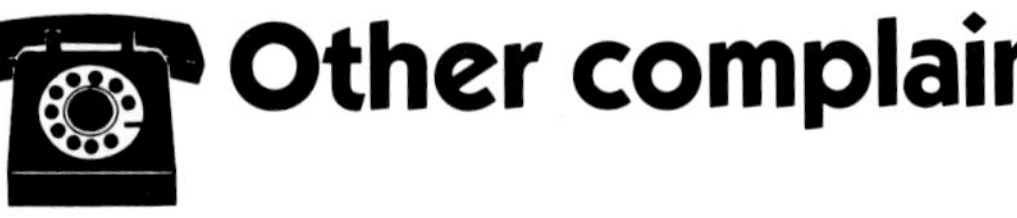

Other complaints

Complaints about nursing homes

The **Nursing Home Ombudsman's** office will handle complaints against nursing homes from patients, relatives, or other concerned people.

Nursing Home Ombudsman
Executive Office of Elder Affairs
38 Chauncy Street
Boston, MA 02111
(617) **727-7273**

The **Division of Health Care Quality** is the office responsible for licensing, certifying, and inspecting nursing homes. They will investigate complaints.

Division of Health Care Quality
Department of Public Health
150 Tremont Street, 2nd floor
Boston, MA 02111
(617) **727-6240**

Complaints about the apartment or house you rent. See pp. 48-49.

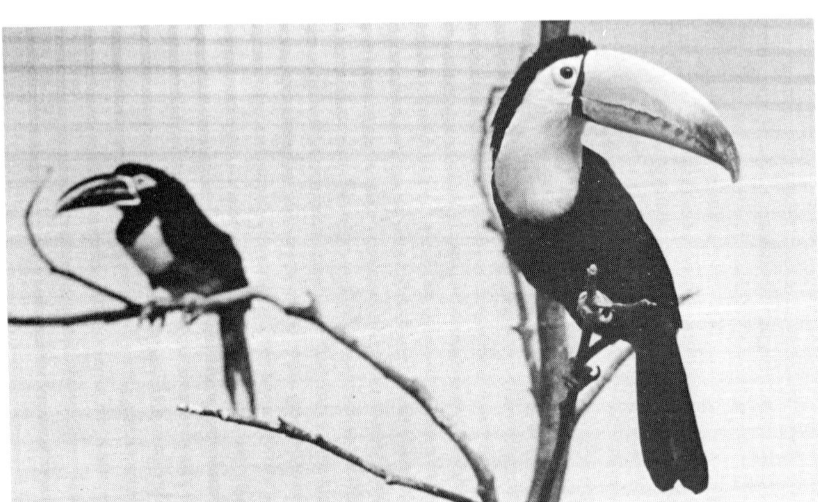

Capron Park Zoo
Attleboro (617) 222-3047

The park includes a tropical rain forest and an Art Museum. See No. 17, p.65.

Complaints about Medicare

Medicare medical insurance complaints

Blue Cross-Blue Shield can explain a bill, tell you whether a claim has been paid, and advise you about your eligibility for a service. There are also Blue Cross-Blue Shield Customer Service offices throughout the state. Look under Blue Cross-Blue Shield in the white pages of your phone book.

If any Medicare claim you submit is disallowed, you will be notified of the reasons by Blue Cross-Blue Shield in writing.

Within 6 months of the date of this notice, you have to make a written request for review if you want to formally disagree. Your letter should tell why you are dissatisfied with the decision. Give your name and health insurance claim number and any other claim number shown on the original notice of decision. Also, provide any other evidence you can to back up your claim.

To decide if the original decision was correct, Blue Cross-Blue Shield will examine the evidence originally submitted plus any additional evidence you have supplied. You do not have an opportunity to appear personally; therefore, the review and second decision will be based only on the written documents. If you are still dissatisfied with the decision, you may request a hearing with Blue Cross-Blue Shield. The request must be made within 6 months of the review decision, and the amount of money in question must be at least $100.

Medicare
Blue Cross-Blue Shield of Massachusetts
100 Summer St.
Boston, MA 02110
1-800-882-1228 (toll free)

Or, if you have a complaint *about* Blue Cross-Blue Shield, you can call:

Massachusetts Division of Insurance
100 Cambridge St.
Boston, MA 02202
(617) **727-3341** or (413) **732-4055** (Springfield)

Medicare hospital insurance complaints

If you are dissatisfied with a denial of payment for services covered by Medicare hospital insurance, the entire appeal will be handled by Social Security.

1. Call or go to any Social Security office. The representative will explain the provisions of Medicare law on which the decision was based.
2. If still dissatisfied, you may request a reconsideration of your claim. If *all* of your claim is denied, you may request a reconsideration within 60 days of the date of this notice. If *part* of your claim is denied, you will receive two notices explaining which services could not be covered and which benefits are paid. Your request for reconsideration must be made in writing no later than 60 days from the date you receive the *second* notice.

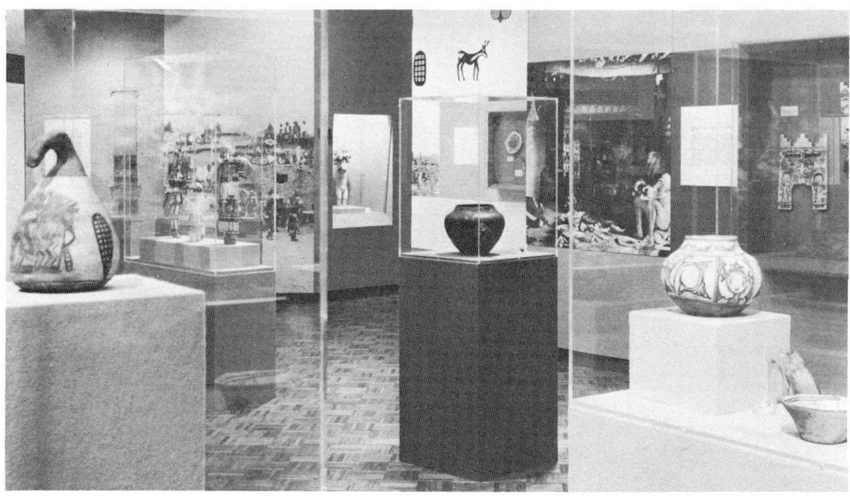

The Museum of Our National Heritage
Lexington (617) 861-6559

A museum of American history with frequently changing exhibits and weekend events. See No. 45, p.67.

3. Medicare claims-reviewers will make a new decision on your claim by considering all written evidence.
   Special note: If a hospital insurance claim is denied because the services you received were not medically necessary, and you had no way of knowing that they were not covered, you can still receive payment.
4. If you are still dissatisfied and the amount in question is $100 or more, you may request a hearing within 60 days from the date of the reconsideration notice. The request has to be in writing on special forms available at any Social Security office. You will be notified at least 10 days before the hearing, and you may have someone represent you or have witnesses testify.

Complaints about Social Security

If you are unhappy about any decisions made by Social Security, these are the steps (in sequence) that you can take:

1. Ask the Social Security Administration to reconsider its decision.
2. If you disagree with that decision, ask for a hearing by an administrative law judge.
3. Request a review by the Social Security Appeals Council.
4. If all else fails, take your case to the federal courts.

There is no charge for any of the appeals before the Social Security Administration.

You can have someone represent you on Social Security matters

You have a right to be represented in any business with Social Security by a person of your choice, but your representative can*not* sign your application for benefits. You appoint this person by filling out a special form, "Appointment of Representative."

If you are paying a fee for your representative's services, it has to be approved by the Social Security Administration. It is against the law for someone to charge a fee that has not been authorized by Social Security; this is to protect you against being overcharged.

Who pays? If your representative is not a lawyer and there are no past benefits due you, you are responsible for paying the fee. However, if your representative is an attorney and there are past-due benefits payable to you, Social Security will pay 25% of the total past-due benefits directly to the attorney.

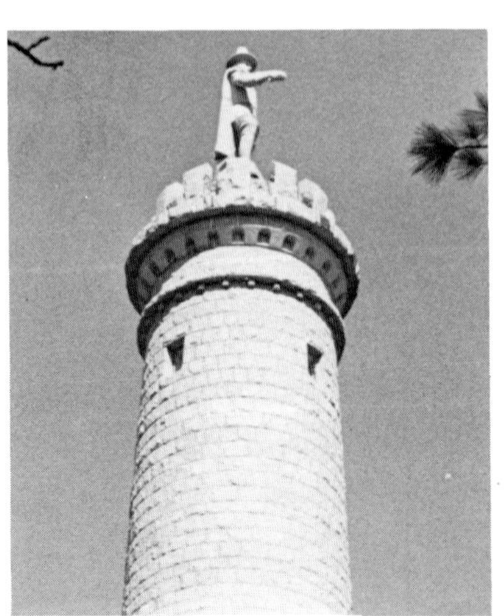

◂ **Myles Standish Monument**
Duxbury

At the center of the Standish Monument State Park, the pilgrim soldier tops a granite tower.

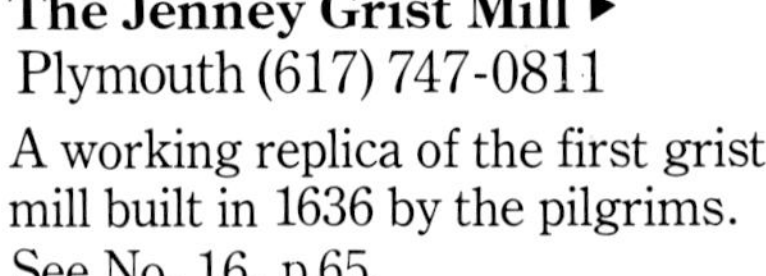

The Jenney Grist Mill ▸
Plymouth (617) 747-0811

A working replica of the first grist mill built in 1636 by the pilgrims. See No. 16, p.65.

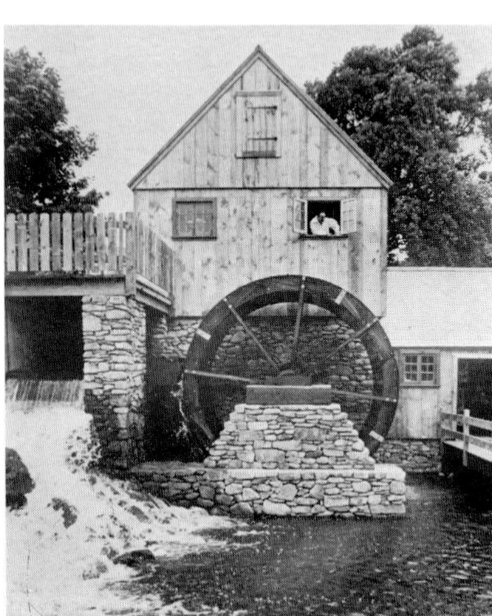

Protecting yourself and your home

Elder abuse and neglect

A recent state law protects all people age 60 and over, living in any Massachusetts community, from "acts or omissions resulting in serious physical or serious emotional injury." Protection is against both abuse and neglect by caretakers.

Under the law, certain people *must* report elder abuse or be subject to a fine. These include: physicians, nurses, family counselors, police, and people in a number of other categories.

But anyone—including the abused or neglected person—*may* report elder abuse and expect to get help.

To report abuse:

Elder Abuse Hotline: **1-800-922-2275** (toll free)

For more information:

Elder Protective Services Program
Executive Office of Elder Affairs
38 Chauncy Street
Boston, MA 02111
(617) **727-7273**
1-800-922-2275 (toll free)

How to protect yourself from crime

If you worry about having your wallet or purse stolen, being attacked by someone while you're out walking, or simply being harassed, there are several steps you can take to reduce your odds of becoming a victim:

- Go for walks when it is light outside, not when it is dark.
- If you must walk at night, go with others and choose busy streets.
- Keep your key where you can reach it quickly, and have it ready before you get to your front door.
- Put your wallet in a *front* pocket—out of a pickpocket's grasp.
- Use a small shoulder purse and wear it so that it opens toward you.
- Police suggest that you carry a whistle where you can use it immediately if you are being threatened.
- Noise scares attackers away, so scream, yell, or whistle to attract help.

How to protect your home

Most people don't need a burglar alarm to make their house or apartment more secure. Getting into the habit of being careful is the cheapest and most effective way to discourage a burglar. Here are a few tips on keeping unwanted "collectors" out of your home:

- Your "secret" key shouldn't be under the mat or over the door, because that is where a

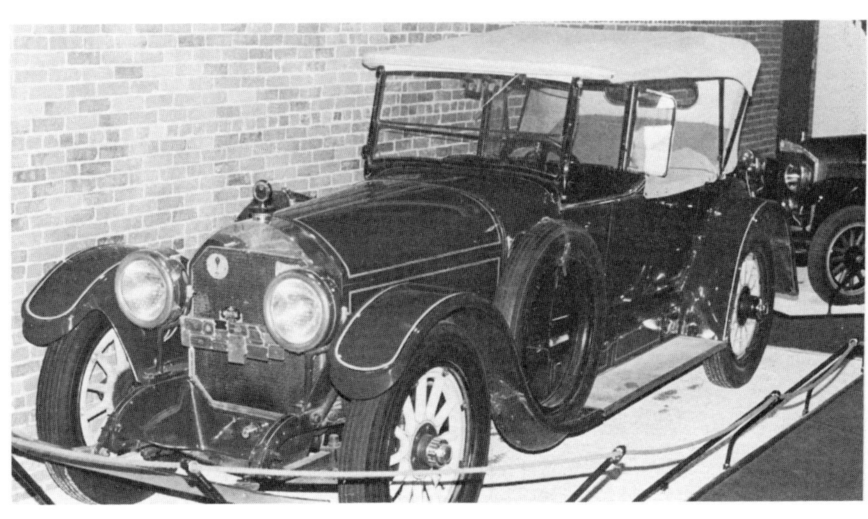

The Museum of Transportation
Brookline (617) 522-6140
350 years of Boston transportation. Seen here, General John "Black Jack" Pershing's custom-built 1918 Locomobile. See No. 28, p.66.

burglar would look first. Give an extra key to a trusted neighbor instead.

- Never leave your doors or windows unlocked and, if possible, have a locksmith install high quality locks. If you care about your things, a good lock is a better investment than insurance.
- Timers for lights are good for when you are away all day or on vacation. Burglars don't want to be seen.
- Dogs are more than good company. An alert dog which barks at strangers usually keeps a burglar from choosing your home.
- Having an identification tag on your key ring or holder is an open invitation to rob your house if the keys are lost.

How to protect yourself from fraud and high pressure sales tactics

Watch out for those who play on your hopes or fears. Watch out for salespeople who argue that a specific opportunity can't wait, that their offer is a limited one, or that time is running out and you should sign now. Take the time to check them out.

The most common frauds are:

Claims for easy health cures, "astounding discoveries" for the treatment of illness, especially for arthritis, rheumatism, or cancer.

Claims for extra income, easy work that promises that you will get rich quick for a cash down payment.

Mail order land developers. If you want to buy a retirement home in the sun, check the company out with a lawyer before you sign anything.

Also, you should see a lawyer before you sign an important contract, such as with a home improvement contractor. Read the fine print and ask for names of satisfied customers you can talk to. See p. 52 for how to find a lawyer.

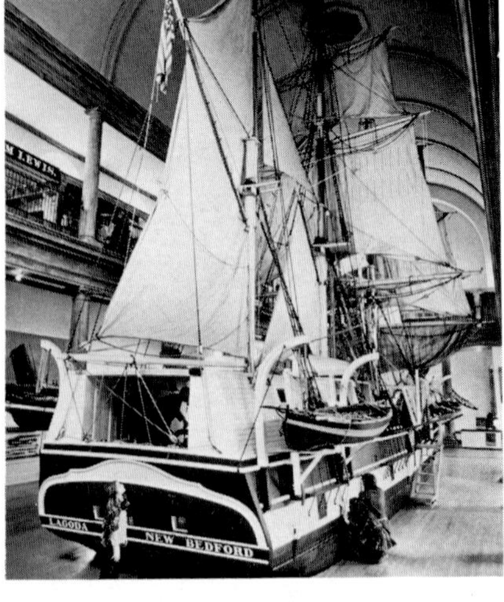

▲ **The Whaling Museum**
New Bedford (617) 997-0046

Half scale replica of the square rigged whaler Lagoda. See No. 7, p.65.

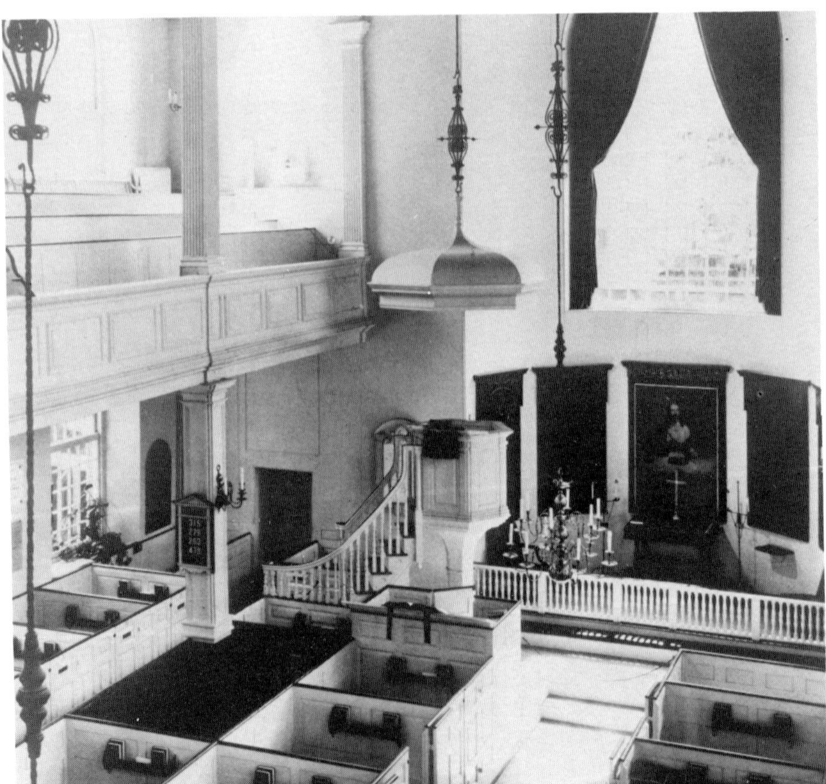

◀ **Old North Church**
Boston (617) 523-6676

Interior of the church, dating from 1724, famous for the tower lanterns: "One if by land; two if by sea."
See No. 30, p.66.

Two Special Places In Your Community

Your senior center

If your area has a Senior Center, it may be an excellent place for you to call or stop by to get information, meet people, and get involved in activities that interest you. Your council on aging or town or city hall should be able to tell you about the senior centers in your community.

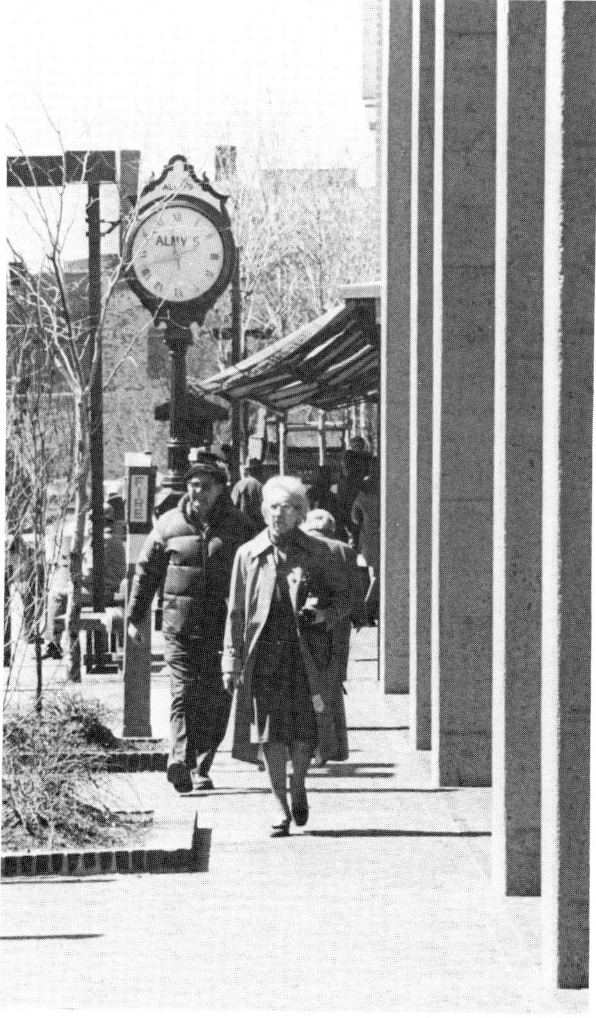

Your council on aging

As we mentioned at the beginning of the book, most cities and towns in Massachusetts have a local council on aging which can give you up-to-date information about programs, discounts, activities, organizations, and many more things of interest to you. A council is a group of local residents dedicated to helping older people in the community. Some councils have staff who will help you, while others rely only on volunteers. In either case, your local council may be the most helpful place for you to turn to for information.

There are councils on aging in more than 330 cities and towns. Those in the 50 largest communities are listed in the next two pages. **If your community isn't listed,** call your city or town hall and ask for the number.

Councils on aging in larger cities and towns*

If your community is not listed here, call your town or city hall.

Arlington—643-6700, ext. 357
Jarvis House
50 Pleasant Street
Arlington, MA 02174

Attleboro—222-9610, ext. 331
City Hall Annex
25 South Main
Attleboro, MA 02703

Belmont—484-7053
Town Hall
455 Concord Avenue
Belmont, MA 02178

Beverly—927-7025
Gar Hall
8 Dana Street
Beverly, MA 01915

*As of April 1985

Boston—725-4366
722-4646 (hotline)
(Mayor's Commission on Affairs of the Elderly)
City Hall
Boston, MA 02201

Braintree—848-1870, ext. 134 or **144**
71 Cleveland Avenue
Braintree, MA 02184

Brockton—583-4163
234 Main Street
Brockton, MA 02401

Brookline—731-8100
O'Shea House
61 Park Street
Brookline, MA 02146

Cambridge—498-9039
51 Inman Street
Cambridge, MA 02139

Chicopee—534-3698
Valley View Senior Center
7 Valley View Court
Chicopee, MA 01020

Danvers—777-0001, ext. 258
12 Sylvan Street
(across from Town Hall)
Danvers, MA 01923

Dedham—326-1650
Dedham Town Hall, lower level
Bryant Street
Dedham, MA 02026

Everett—387-7100
90 Chelsea Street
Everett, MA 02149

Fall River—675-6011, ext. 293
One Government Center
Fall River, MA 02722

Fitchburg—345-9598
Senior Citizens Center
14 Wallace Avenue
Fitchburg, MA 01420

Framingham—620-4819
Callahan Senior Center
154 Pearl Street
Framingham, MA 01701

Gloucester—283-0043
Mayor's Office
Gloucester, MA 01930

Haverhill—374-2390
10 Welcome Street
Haverhill, MA 01830

Holyoke—534-2208
310 Appleton Street
Holyoke, MA 01040

Lawrence—688-8451
155 Haverhill Street
Lawrence, MA 01841

Leominster—537-1569
Senior Citizens Drop-In Center
39 Mechanic Street
Leominster, MA 01453

Lexington—861-0194
1475 Massachusetts Avenue
Lexington, MA 02173

Lowell—459-7971
400 Merrimack Street
Lowell, MA 01852

Lynn—599-0110
Greater Lynn Senior Services
90 Exchange Street
Lynn, MA 01901

Malden—324-6600, ext. 195
Malden City Hall
200 Pleasant Street
Malden, MA 02148

Marlboro—485-6492
Community Center
250 Main Street
Marlboro, MA 01752

Medford—396-6010
101 Riverside Avenue
Medford, MA 02155

Melrose—665-4304
City Hall - 562 Main Street
Melrose, MA 02176

Methuen—794-3296
77 Lowell Street
Methuen, MA 01844

Milton—698-0100, ext. 247
Milton Town Office Building
525 Canton Avenue
Milton, MA 02186

Natick—655-5334
Natick Senior Center
10 Wilson Street
Natick, MA 01760

Needham—444-5100, ext. 116
83 Pickering Street
Needham, MA 02192

New Bedford—990-2000
758 Purchase Street
P.O. Box F658
New Bedford, MA 02740

Newton—552-7170
Newton City Hall
1000 Commonwealth Avenue
Newton, MA 02159

Northampton—586-6950, ext. 228
Memorial Hall
240 Main Street
Northampton, MA 01060

Norwood—762-1201
165 Nahatan Street
Norwood, MA 02062

Peabody—531-2254
75 Central Street
Peabody, MA 01960

Pittsfield—447-7374
Senior Center
33 Bradford Street
Pittsfield, MA 01201

Quincy—773-1380, ext. 243, 245, or **457**
1120 Hancock Street
Quincy, MA 02169

Revere—284-3600, ext. 170
Revere City Hall
281 Broadway
Revere, MA 02151

Salem—744-0924
5 Broad Street
Salem, MA 01970

Somerville—625-6600, ext. 236 or **237**
City Hall
1 Davis Square
Somerville, MA 02144

Springfield—787-6124
City Hall, Room 4
36 Court Street
Springfield, MA 01103

Taunton—823-6911
30 Olney Street
Taunton, MA 02780

Wakefield—245-3312
Lincoln Schoolhouse
26 Crescent Street
Wakefield, MA 01880

Waltham—899-7228
174 Moody Street
Waltham, MA 02154

Watertown—924-6370
Town Hall
149 Main Street
Watertown, MA 02172

Wellesley—235-3961
219 Washington Street
Wellesley, MA 02181

West Springfield—781-7750, ext. 3264 or **3265**
128 Park Street
West Springfield, MA 01089

Westfield—562-6435
General Shepherd Apartments
40 Main Street
Westfield, MA 01085

Weymouth—335-2000, ext. 50 or **55**
Jefferson School Building
200 Middle Street
Weymouth, MA 02190

Woburn—933-0700, ext. 22
City Hall
10 Common Street
Woburn, MA 01801

Worcester—791-7286
425 Pleasant Street
Worcester, MA 01609
(Ask for their local services directory, "Informational Guide.")

Some Organizations to Join

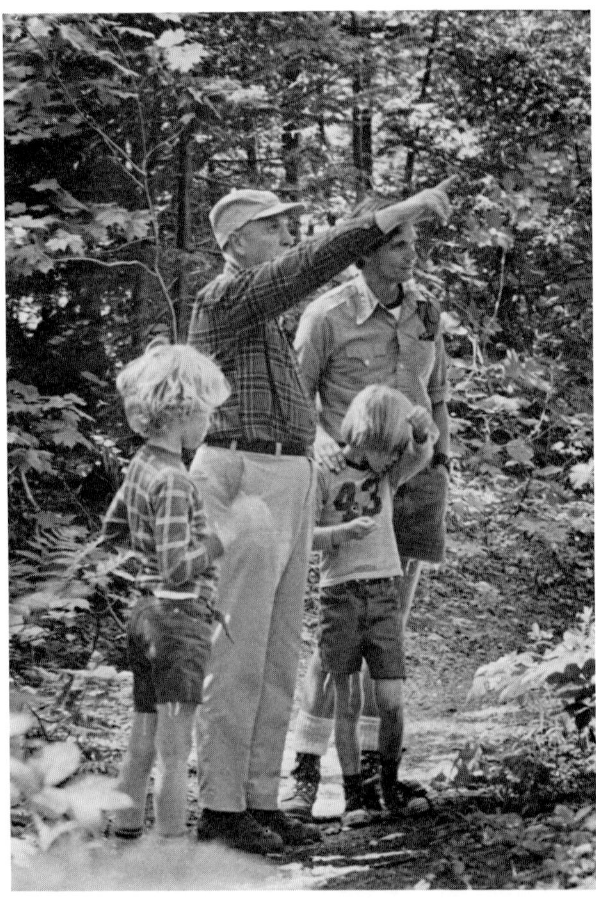

Appalachian Mountain Club guide points out a natural curiosity.

It's often been observed that America is a land of organizations. Whatever your interest, there's an organization to join, from collectors' clubs and hobby groups, to service organizations, to organizations dedicated to social change. Here is a small sampling:

Massachusetts Association of Older Americans
110 Arlington Street
Boston, MA 02116
(617) **426-0805**

$4/yr. individual membership. Bi-monthly newsletter. Special events, education and training in advocacy skills.

Massachusetts Audubon Society
South Great Road
Lincoln, MA 01773
(617) **259-9500**

$20/yr. individual membership. 60+ senior membership $10/yr. Monthly newsletter, annual yearbook, discounts on courses, programs, special events, free use of sanctuaries.

Massachusetts Horticultural Society
Membership Department
300 Mass. Ave.
Boston, MA 02115
(617) **536-9280**

$35/yr. individual membership. Quarterly newsletter. Courses, programs, special events.

Appalachian Mountain Club
5 Joy Street
Boston, MA 02158
(617) **523-0636**

23-69 yrs: $30/yr. + $5 to join. 70+, senior member: $20/yr. + $5 to join. Activities, publications.

League of Women Voters of Massachusetts
8 Winter Street
Boston, MA 02108
(617) **357-8380**

Nonpartisan political action. Membership open to men and women. Town or city Leagues set meetings and dues.

New England Historic Geneological Society
101 Newbury Street
Boston, MA 02116
(617) **536-5740**

$40/yr. individual membership. Use of library, special programs and lectures, quarterly journal, book loan available to members by mail, monthly newsletter.

American Automobile Association (AAA)
AAA of Massachusetts
1050 Hingham Street
Rockland, MA 02370

AAA auto clubs in several areas; membership fees vary. Emergency road service; motor travel service (maps, tour books, trip planning, etc.); full service travel agency; discounts on Avis and Hertz car rentals and used car sales, General Cinema, Showcase, and Sack movie tickets; free credit card registration service; insurance at group rates; other benefits.

Rockland	(617) **871-5980**
Boston	(617) **723-0800**
Lawrence	(617) **681-9200**
Worcester	(617) **853-7000**
Springfield	(413) **785-1381**
Holyoke	(413) **539-9881**
Pittsfield	(413) **445-5635**

American Association of Retired Persons
AARP
823 Park Square Building
Boston, MA 02116
(617) **426-1185**

$5/yr. individual or married couple's membership. Membership open only to people 50 and over. Bimonthly magazines, monthly newsletter, free booklets, discounts, special insurance offer, pharmacy service by mail.

Gray Panthers National Headquarters
3700 Chestnut Street
Philadelphia, PA 19104
(215) **382-3300**

Activist, intergenerational group combatting age discrimination, with a media watch project and current emphasis on health care and peace. Membership dues based on ability to pay. Contact the group in your part of the state for more information.

Gray Panthers of Greater Boston
11 Garden Street
Cambridge, MA 02138
(617) **497-5767**

Gray Panthers of the Pioneer Valley
P.O. Box 771
Amherst, MA 01004
(413) **549-7273**

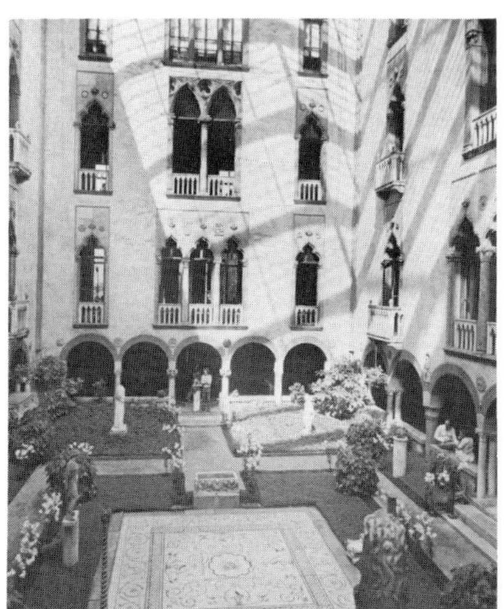

◂ **Isabella Stewart Gardner Museum**
Boston (617) 734-1359

Seasonally planted courtyard of Isabella Stewart Gardner's Italian Renaissance style mansion that houses an excellent painting and decorative arts collection. Evening concerts. See No. 23, p.66.

Springfield Armory Museum ▸
Springfield (413) 734-8551

The world's largest small arms collection, managed by the National Park Service. See No. 67, p.69.

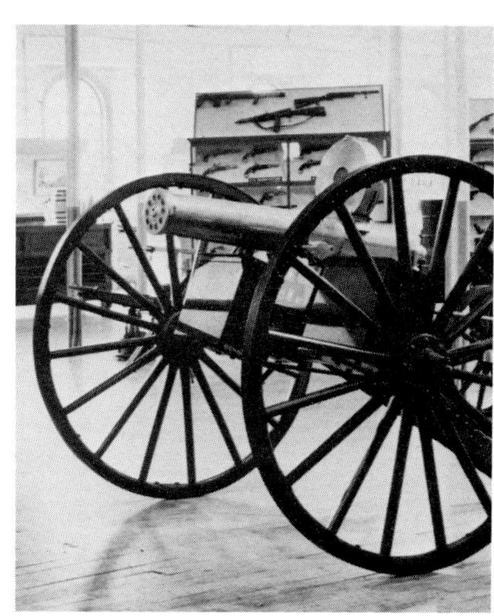

Things to Read and Watch

The man who does not read good books has no advantage over the man who can't read them.
—Mark Twain

Believe it or not, there are many more magazines and books about life after 60 than we have listed here. Your senior center or local library may have many of the books, as well as subscriptions to the periodicals.

Magazines and other periodicals

Aging *$15.00; 6 issues/year*
Superintendent of Documents
Government Printing Office
Washington, D.C. 02402
Published by the U.S. Department of Health and Human Services.

Boston Seniority *free for age 60+; 12 issues/year*
Mayor's Commission on Affairs of the Elderly
(617) 722-4646; distributed at senior centers.

A publication for Boston residents.

Elder Affairs *free; 12 issues/year*
Massachusetts Executive Office of Elder Affairs
Boston, MA
727-8931 in Boston area, or 1-800-882-2003 (toll free) outside Boston area.

Newsletter of the Massachusetts Executive Office of Elder Affairs. Up-to-date information.

50 Plus *$15.00; 12 issues/year*
99 Garden Street
Marion, Ohio 43302

New England Senior Citizen *$9.95; 12 issues/year*
470 Boston Post Rd.
Weston, MA 02193

Newspaper format, variety of articles. Distributed free at senior centers; also by paid subscription.

Gerontopics *$16.00; 4 issues/year*
New England Gerontology Center, Durham, NH
Human Sciences Press
72 Fifth Avenue
New York, NY 10011

Modern Maturity *$5.00; 6 issues/year*
AARP (American Association of Retired Persons)
1909 K Street, N.W.
Washington, D.C. 20049

An excellent source of information. Comes with membership.

The Older American *$4.00; 6 issues/year*
MAOA (Massachusetts Association of Older Americans)
110 Arlington Street
Boston, MA 02116
(617) 426-0805

A good investment for Massachusetts residents. Has information about state programs, policy changes, and interesting news items.

Senior Advocate *$5.00; 24 issues/year*
340 Main St., Room 551
Worcester, MA 01608

Free at senior centers; also by paid subscription.

United Retirement Bulletin *$21.00, 12 issues/yr.*
United Business Service
210 Newbury Street
Boston, MA 02116

Health, taxes, travel, financial information

Local Newsletters—your local council on aging may publish a newsletter that would be of interest to you (see pp. 81-83 for how to reach your council).

Your local newspaper

More and more newspapers are giving special attention to things that affect and are of interest to people 60 and over. Some, such as the *Boston Globe* and *Boston Herald*, have a special column and a reporter who specializes in this. If your own paper isn't covering things that you would like to know more about, you might suggest that they put in more items of interest to older people.

Some books of special interest that might change your life

Retirement Book—Joan Adler
***Going Like Sixty**—Richard Armor
How To Retire Successfully—Shirley Ashton
The Complete Retirement Planning Book—Peter Dickinson
The Best Years Book—Hugh Downs and Richard Roll
***It Takes a Long Time To Become Young**—Garson Kanin
Maggie Kuhn on Aging—Margaret Kuhn (leader of "Gray Panthers")
Success Over Sixty—Albert Myers and Christopher Anderson
Aging, the Fulfillment of Life—Henri Nouwen and Walter Gaffney
Aging Is Not for Sissies—Terry Schuckman

Moving and travel

Sunbelt Retirement—Peter Dickinson
Where To Retire on a Small Income—Norman Ford
Now It's Your Turn To Travel—Rosalind Massow

Expert advice

A Good Age—Alex Comfort
Fires of Autumn—Peter Dickinson
***Successful Aging**—Olga Knopf
The 36-Hour Day—Nancy Mace and Peter Rabins
Love in the Later Years: the Emotional, Physical, Sexual, and Social Potential of the Elderly—James A. Peterson & Barbara Payne
***Sixty-Plus and Fit Again**—Magda Rosenberg
Enjoy Old Age—B. F. Skinner and M. E. Vaughan
Getting Older and Staying Young—Dr. D.D. Stonecypher, Jr.
Feeling Alive after Sixty-Five—Robert Taylor, M.D.
Take Care of Yourself: A Consumer's Guide to Medical Care—Donald Vickery and James Fries

Practical matters

***You and Your Will**—Paul Ashley
More Money for Your Retirement—John Barnes
How To Make a Will—Parnell Callahan
Rosefsky's Guide to Financial Security for the Mature Family—Robert Rosefsky

Other books

***Grandparents**—Charlie Shedd
Living in a Nursing Home—Sarah Burger & Martha D'Evasmo
Educational Opportunities of Greater Boston
The Educational Exchange of Greater Boston

THE directory for the Boston area. Probably the best single source of listings of professionals, agencies and organizations that can help solve problems in Boston and 90 surrounding cities and towns is Jonathon Starr's exceptionally well organized *Human Service Yellow Pages of Greater Boston*, available from:

Human Service Yellow Pages
P.O. Box 106
West Somerville, MA 02144
(617) **426-2424** (Call for current price)

*Also published in a Large Print edition.

Tuning in

Radio and television are sources of up-to-date information on many things of special interest. One television program that focuses specially on topics of interest to people 60 and over is "Prime Time" on WBZ-TV, Channel 4, aired Sundays at 8:30 a.m. Your local cable stations may also have programs of particular interest, especially in relation to local events and organizations that serve your area.

Unusual places

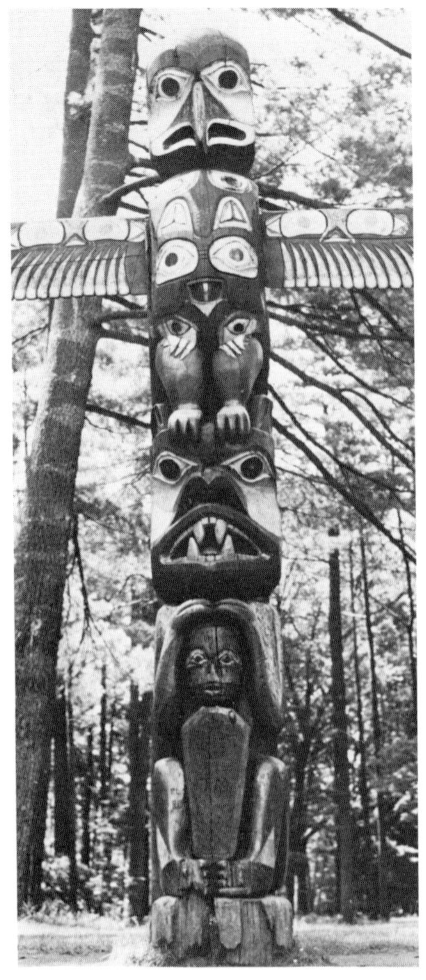

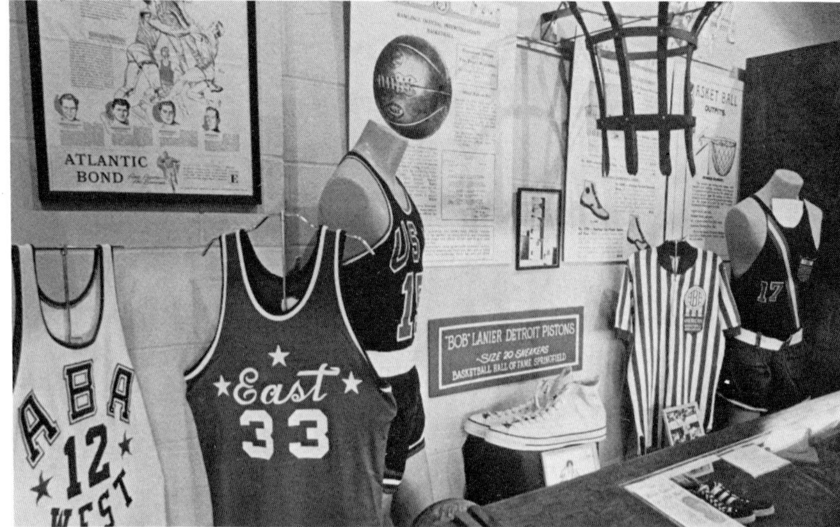

Basketball Hall of Fame
Springfield (413) 781-6500
The history of basketball from its beginning in 1891. See No. 63, p.68.

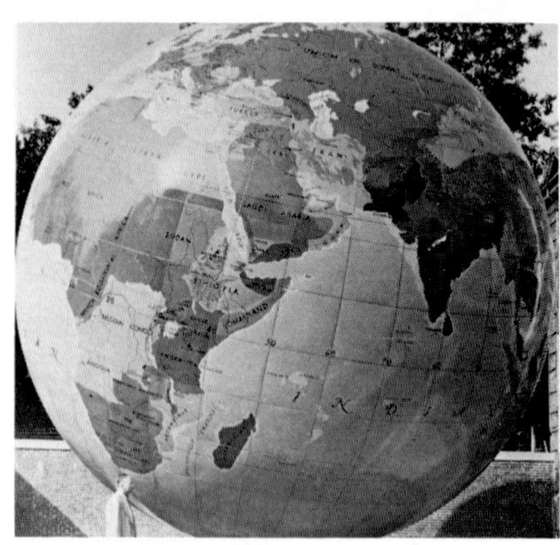

The Giant Globe at Babson College
Wellesley, (617) 235-1200
See No. 43, p.67.

John Woodman Higgins Armory
Worcester (617) 853-6015
Finest collection of armor in the country. See No. 58, p.68.

Hammond Castle
West Gloucester (617) 283-2080
A medieval style castle appropriately furnished. See No. 56, p.68.

Clockwise:
Look Park
Northampton
A totem pole built by Northampton Boy Scouts.

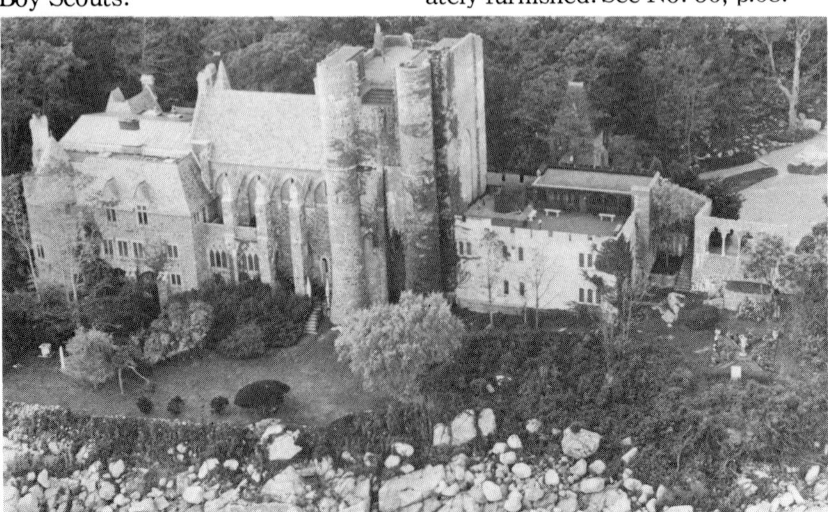

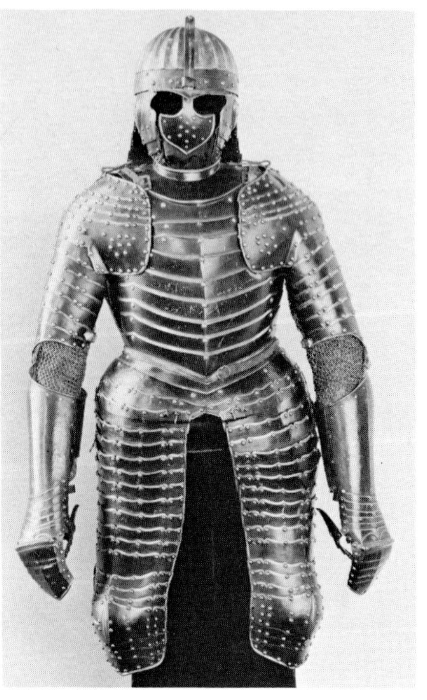

Referral Sources for Your Area

Printed directories

A listing of service organizations in your own area may be available from your local council on aging (see pp. 81-83), your Home Care Corporation (pp. 54-55), or the organization for your area that is listed on this page. Sometimes there is a charge for such a directory; they will tell you when you call.

An especially valuable directory is the *Human Service Yellow Pages of Greater Boston* (see p. 87).

By telephone

The council on aging in your own community (see pp. 81-83) and the Home Care Corporation for your area (see pp. 54-55) are excellent sources of information on many subjects of interest to you. And if you live in Boston, don't forget to refer to the "Boston Page" in this book (p. 90).

In addition, the infomation and referral services listed below should be helpful in directing you to useful resources in your area. Call the one nearest you.

Amherst Area (Hampshire Country)	**Direct Information Service** Jones Library	**(413) 256-0121** **1-800-282-7779** (toll free)
Boston Area	**Information and Referral Service** United Way of Massachusetts Bay	(617) **482-1454**
Brockton Area	**Brockton Area Help Line**	(617) **584-4357**
Fall River Area	**Info-Line**	(617) **674-1100**
Greenfield Area	**Social Service Help** Franklin Community Action Corp.	(413) **774-2318** **1-800-322-0270** (toll free)
Hyannis Area	**Cape Cod Community Council**	(617) **775-0464** **1-800-462-8002** (toll free)
Lawrence Area	**Answers** Memorial Hall Library, Andover	(617) **470-1184**
Lynn Area (North Shore)	**Information and Referral Service** United Way of Massachusetts Bay	(617) **599-6800**
Marlboro Area	**Together, Inc.**	(617) **485-2424**
North Adams Area (Northern Berkshire County)	**Help Line, Inc.**	(413) **664-6391**
Pittsfield Area (Central and south Berkshire County	**Berkshire United Way**	(413) **442-6940** **1-800-251-5300** (toll free)
Springfield Area (Hampden County)	**FIRST CALL** United Way of Pioneer Valley	(413) **737-2712**
Worcester Area	**First Call** United Way of Central Mass.	(617) **755-1233**

Boston Page

Older residents of Boston have a wide variety of services available. The Commission on Affairs of the Elderly, the city's council on aging, provided the following listing of important numbers to call.

Information & Referral:

Central Office	**725-4366**
Elderly Hotline	**722-4646**

Community Services/Senior Shuttle (van):

Neighborhood Offices:

Allston-Brighton	**254-6191**
Ashmont/Fields Corner	**436-0736**
Back Bay/Beacon Hill	**725-4369**
Bowdoin/Uphams Corner/ Lower Mills	**436-0736**
Charlestown	**725-3984**
East Boston	**725-3986**
Fenway/Mission Hill	**725-4369**
Jamaica Plain	**325-5060**
Mattapan	**427-1743**
North End	**725-3986**
Roslindale	**325-5060**
Roxbury	**427-1743**
South Boston	**725-3984**
South End	**725-4369**
W. Roxbury/Hyde Park	**364-9308**

Employment/Volunteer	**725-3987**
R.S.V.P. (see p. 37)	**725-3988**
Senior Aides (see p. 31)	**725-3989**
Health Services:	
Bright Eyes (eye exam) **Blood Pressure Screening** **Sound Screen** (hearing exam)	**725-4050 or 725-4486**
Nursing Home Ombudsman	**725-3983**
Government Benefits	**725-3958**
Senior Clubs Information	**725-4373**
Boston Seniority (free paper)	**725-3719 or 725-3716**
Public Information/Legislation	**725-4360**
Emergency Numbers:	
Police	**911**
Fire	**911**
Ambulance	**911**
Mayor's 24-hour Service	**725-4000**

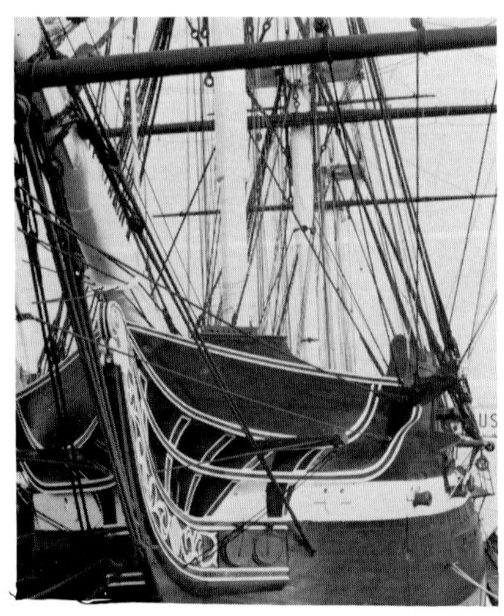

◀ **U.S.S. Constitution**
Boston (617) 242-0543

"Old Ironsides," restored to its original fighting condition for the War of 1812. See No. 37, p.67.

Christian Science Center ▶
Boston (617) 262-2300, ext. 3795

The famous maparium (which allows you to stand inside a stained glass globe), the Mother Church and the publishing center are part of a free tour of the Center. No. 19, p.66.

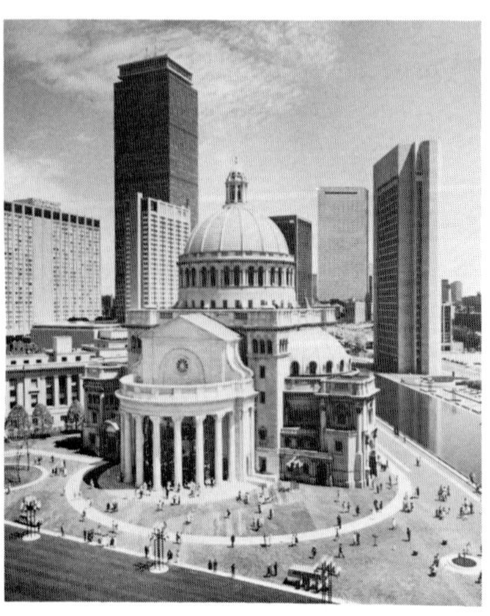

Did We Miss Something?

Since we probably haven't thought of everything you might want to know, here's a list of offices that you can write or call for more information. Generally these offices are open Monday through Friday from 9 to 5. They are waiting to hear from you.

For Everyone

Many subjects	**Massachusetts Executive Office of Elder Affairs** 38 Chauncy Street Boston, MA 02111	**727-8931** "Elder Hot Line" if you live in Boston area or **1-800-882-2003** (toll-free) if you live outside Boston area (Mon-Fri, 9-5)
Many subjects	**Massachusetts Association of Older Americans** 110 Arlington Street Boston, MA 02116	(617) **426-0804** (Mon-Fri, 8:30-4)
Many Subjects	**Council on Aging** in your own city or town (your town or city hall will have the address)	Telephone: (look up the numbers on 81-83, or call your town or city hall)
Many subjects Eastern Mass. only	**Information and Referral** United Way of Massachusetts Bay 87 Kilby Street Boston, MA 02109	(617) **482-1454**
State government and programs	**Citizen Information Service** Office of the Secretary of State One Ashburton Place Boston, MA 02108	(617) **727-7030** if you live in Boston area *or* **1-800-392-6090** (toll free) if you live outside Boston area
Employment	**Massachusetts Executive Office of Economic Affairs** Hurley Building Boston, MA 02114	**1-800-882-JOBS** (toll free)
Voter Information and government services	**Voter Information Phone** Massachusetts League of Women Voters 8 Winter Street Boston, MA 02111	(617) **357-5880** if you live in Boston area *or* **1-800-882-1649** (toll-free) if you live outside Boston area

For Boston Residents

Many subjects	**Mayor's Commission on Affairs of the Elderly** City Hall Boston, MA 02201	"Elderly Hotline" **722-4646**

If you write, a simple postcard will do. But *be sure you write down your own name and full address* so they can get back in touch with you.

Ten Important Phone Numbers

Look up the numbers and fill them in here for easy reference.

Number	Contact
____________	**Council on Aging**
____________	**Police Department**
____________	**Fire Department**
____________	**Doctor**
____________	**Lawyer**
____________	**Town or City Hall**
____________	**Social Security Office**
722-4646	**"Elderly Hotline" for Boston Residents**
727-8931	**"Elder Hot Line"** (Mass. Elder Affairs) Boston area
1-800-882-2003	(toll free) if you live outside Boston area
727-7030	**Citizen Information Service** Boston area
1-800-392-6090	(toll free) if you live outside Boston area

Other telephone numbers for information or assistance

You may have overlooked the "Self-help Guide" that is included in the front of the Boston white pages telephone book. From page 2 through page 5 there is an extensive list of "Community Service Numbers" that you may find useful for contacting a variety of government and non-profit organizations in Boston, Brookline, Cambridge, and Somerville. If you live elsewhere, look for a similar section in the telephone directory for your own area.

For additional copies of this book

If you are missing the information flyer about ordering additional copies, or if you want more detail about quantity discounts or personalized covers, please contact the publisher:

Center for Information Sharing
77 North Washington Street
Boston, MA 02114
(617) 742-3222

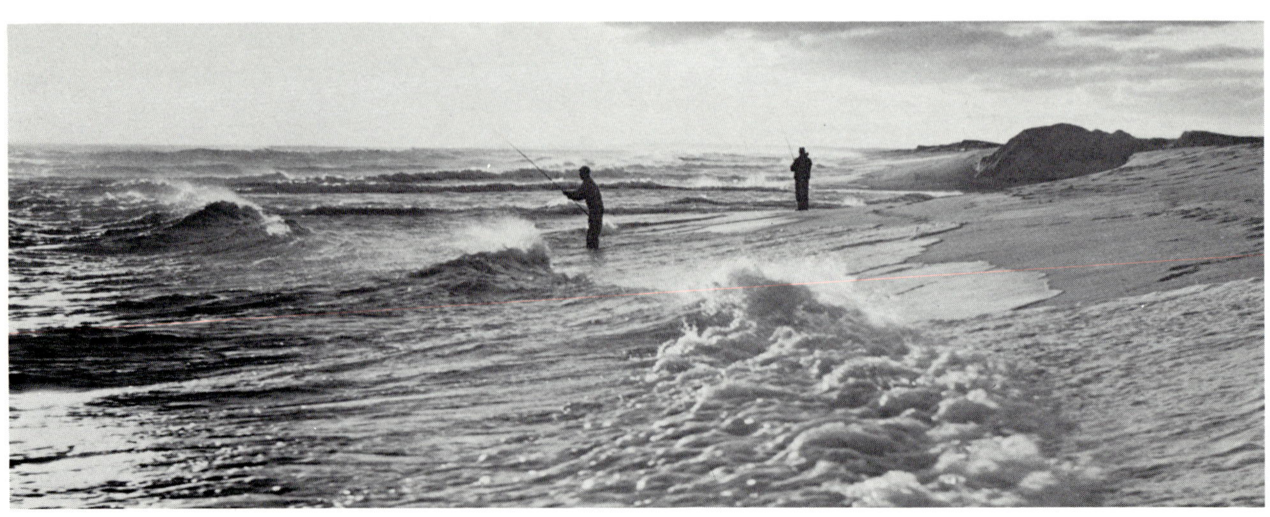